S0-AGW-791

The Science of Meditation, Yoga, and Prayer

Amitava Dasgupta, Ph.D.

The Science of Meditation, Yoga, and Prayer

Published by Blue River Press
Indianapolis, Indiana
www.brpressbooks.com

Distributed by Cardinal Publishers Group
Tom Doherty Company, Inc.
www.cardinalpub.com

ISBN:987-1-68157-021-1

Author: Amitava Dasgupta, Ph.D.
Editor: Dani McCormick
Cover Design: David Miles
Interior Design: Dave Reed

Published: 2017

Printed in the United States of America

The Science of Meditation, Yoga, and Prayer

Contents

Tables

Preface

Yoga represents a system of movement and breathing exercises intended to foster mind-body connection. Yoga, an ancient practice originating from India, was introduced by several popular yoga teachers (gurus) in the West between the 1930s and the 1970s. Currently, yoga is extremely popular and trendy with approximately 15.8 million Americans practicing yoga today. Many yoga practitioners also meditate on a regular basis as the two practices are often incorporated together.

There are many books on yoga and the spiritual practice of meditation. This book is not intended to teach readers yoga or how to meditate. The objective of this book is to convince readers to practice yoga and/or meditation because there are many physical and mental health benefits associated with such practice. Although exercise has many health benefits, scientific studies indicate that yoga and meditation are superior to exercise alone. Moreover, exercise stimulates the sympathetic nervous system, but yoga stimulates the para-sympathetic nervous system thus providing mental calmness, reduced blood pressure, and many other additional health benefits. In addition, risk of injury is higher from an exercise protocol than practicing yoga.

All physical and mental health benefits of yoga and meditation described in this book are backed by rigorous scientific research. At the end of the book, I have provided a list of scientific papers published in reputed, peer reviewed medical journals so that readers may also read original scientific papers for more information. Today some physicians are recommending yoga and meditation in addition to standard medicine. There is an overwhelming amount of scientific evidence that yoga is an effective complementary and integrative health approach for reducing stress, depression, and anxiety. Yoga is also effective in reducing lower back pain, pain associated with several diseases, symptoms of menopause, and insomnia. Moreover, yoga enhances cardiovascular function, reduces anxiety, depression, and chronic pain, and improves sleep pattern, overall well-being, and quality of life. Yoga is effective in preventing alcohol and drug abuse. Meditation also has similar physical and mental health benefits. The practice of meditation is even very effective in increasing mental power and concentration.

The secondary and accompanying part of this book addresses religion particularly the practice and philosophy of prayer and the potential transformative power prayer can have. Religious practices date back 500,000 years in human history and religiosity/spirituality also contributes to overall well-being of individuals. However, individuals who participate in religious practices such as attending religious services get more mental health benefits from religion than individuals who passively belong to a religious group but do not participate in religious services. Sometimes prayers are answered but no one knows scientific mechanism by which some prayers are answered. Nevertheless, papers published in scientific journals indicate that prayers may have unexpected healing effects on critically ill patients. Moreover, even today with many medical wonders, miracles are still reported in medical journals where a patient who is destined to die miraculously survives. I have personally witnessed one such incidence when all medical interventions failed and my mother was destined to die in June 2011, but miraculously survived when my Christian wife prayed at her bedside (see bonus section). My mother is still alive with no loss of cognitive functions unexplainable from current knowledge of medical science.

In this book I made all attempts to be subjective and everything discussed in this book are backed by rigorous scientific research. I like to thank my wife Alice for putting up with me when I was spending late nights and weekends on the computer to prepare this manuscript. My objective is to convince readers that there are many health benefits of yoga and meditation so that readers who currently do not practice yoga or meditation will be excited to try this alternative health modality for better health and emotional well-being. My hard work will be rewarded if readers enjoy this book.

Respectfully,

Amitava Dasgupta

1
The Origin of Religion, Prayer, and Miracles

Introduction

We live in a technologically advanced society but despite astonishing growth in science and technology approximately 90% of the world population believes in a God and participates in some religious and spiritual practices. Even in a technologically advanced and secular country like the U.S., 83.1% of the population practices some religion (78.4% identified themselves as Christian). Atheism is actually rare throughout the world with more than thirty countries reporting no atheists living in their countries. In Canada, 12.5% of the population is non-religious but only 1.9% are atheist. In the U.S., 16.1% of the population has no religious affiliation but only 1.6% identified themselves as atheist .[1]

Early evidence of religion probably dated back 500,000 years ago when ritual treatment of deceased took place during Paleolithic period. Religion has in part survived for such a long time period in human history because religious beliefs provide amazing coping skills by helping to make sense of sufferings and dealing with the uncertainties of life and afterlife. Religion also promotes good human values, social rules, and facilitates peaceful communal living, cooperation between individual members of the society, and mutual support.

Philosophers, anthropologists, evolutionary biologists, psychiatrists, neurobiologists and other scientists propose various hypotheses attempting to explain origin of religion. Although scientists consider religion as a byproduct of large brain size of humans compared to other animals and attempt to explain religious and or spiritual experiences from complex neurobiological processes thus demystifying religion as a known biological process, philosophers have different perspectives. In this chapter various hypotheses regarding origin of religion are discussed, while in Chapter 3, various approaches discussing religious experiences from complex neuro-biochemical processes is addressed.

Religion: From Prehistoric Times to Modern Times

Archeologists consider intentional burial of prehistoric Homo sapiens 500,000–300,000 years ago as the earliest known evidence of religious rituals. In the prehistoric time, humans lived in small bands as hunters and even at that time there was some primitive religious belief such as worship of ancestor. In the most primitive culture, the basic form of religion was initiated with a belief that spiritual forces exist pervading all creations. It was called "Mana" which was derived from the name given by prehistoric inhabitants of Melanesia. A beautiful tree, a unique rock formation, or even certain animals could be considered containing a higher concentration of spiritual force (Mana). Those objects were worshipped in order to obtain desired effect. The next step of development was "Animism," which taught that spiritual energies are underlying forces for all events and many objects of the physical world may carry some spiritual significance. At that point it was believed that there were two types of sprits; ancestor's spirits and nature's sprits. It was also assumed that nature's spirits can inhibit natural objects of the physical world such as plants, rocks, and lakes. In the next stage of human evolution, religious belief was polytheistic (faith in many gods and goddesses and worship of figurines) .[2]

The development of complex and more organized religions started when humans abandoned hunter-gatherer lifestyle and started farming during Neolithic period (new Stone Age, approximately 11,000 years ago). At that time ancient humans hypothesized that there was a connection between fertility of farmland and fertility of women because role of males in human reproduction was not understood. Therefore, many ancient religions were pagan religions where God was a woman.

Çatalhöyük, Central Anatolia, Turkey is a UNESCO world heritage site where archeological excavation by British archeologist James Mellaart discovered ruins of one of world's most famous ancient Neolithic village where approximately 10,000 inhabitants lived approximately 8,660 years ago. That village was also the spiritual center of Central Anatolia at that time.[3] A striking feature of Çatalhöyük was discovery of its female figurines carved and molded from marble, blue and black limestones, as well as clay and probably represented a female deity.

As humans transitioned from hunter-gatherer to farmers, religion became an important part of civilization. Because farmers were completely dependent on Mother Nature for rain and fertility of land, many religious rituals were developed in order to please gods and goddess in the heaven so that they could send rain on time for successful growing of crops. At that time domestication of animals had started and in order to please gods and goddess animals were sacrificed. In addition, human blood was also used in some rituals including even human sacrifice. Animal sacrifice on certain auspicious days is still practiced in modern religions including Hinduism and Islam.

Writing was important for progress of both civilization and religion. Writing was probably invented in ancient Mesopotamia around 3200 BC. According to pyramid texts from Egypt, one of the oldest written texts on religion approximately around 2400 BC, Egyptians practiced polytheism. Their religion was strongly influenced by tradition, which caused them to resist change. Moreover, Egyptians believed in afterlife and as a result they preserved dead bodies by mummification. In addition, large pyramids were constructed as tombs for the pharaohs because they believed pharaohs became gods after death (Pharaohs were associated with Horus, son of Re, the Sun God).

Ancient religions were mostly polytheistic in nature. Many of the ancient Greek people recognized the major (Olympian) gods and goddesses. Most of the Roman gods and goddesses were a blend of several religious influences including Greek influences and also influences of old religions of the Etruscans or Latin tribes.

An example of such mixed origins was the goddess Diana to whom the Roman King Servius Tullius built the temple on the Aventine Hill. Essentially she was an old Latin goddess from the earliest of times. One of the oldest religions in the world still practiced today as the third most popular religion is Hinduism, which is also a polytheistic religion with a central belief in many gods and goddesses. However, according to the Holy Text of Bhagavad Gita, there is a supreme God Brahman and all gods and goddesses are basically demigods and demigoddesses.

Pantheism (a belief that all is divine or God) has prevailed as a major religious belief in many ancient civilizations. In pantheism, the belief is that God is present everywhere and everything in the cosmos including this material world is divine in nature. Therefore, it is important to live in harmony with nature. Although Hinduism, in general, is considered polytheistic in nature, philosophy of Advaita Vedanta School is in harmony with pantheism. In addition, in some varieties of Kabbalistic Judaism, in Celtic spirituality, and in Sufi mysticism the basic belief system is pantheism. Some new age spirituality is also based on pantheism. Probably Dutch philosopher Spinoza was the first modern day philosopher who clearly introduced pantheistic belief in God.

Spinoza was born in Amsterdam in 1632, into a family of Jewish immigrants and was trained in Talmudic scholarship. However later his philosophy deviated from traditional Jewish belief and he did not become a Rabbi. He earned his living as a humble lens-grinder and died in February 1677. Spinoza believed that everything that exists is God. However, he did not hold the converse view that God is no more than the sum of what exists. God has infinite qualities, of which we can perceive only few. Therefore, God must exist in dimensions far beyond those of the visible world and Spinoza's God is not the conventional Judo-Christian God. Later Einstein was influenced by his philosophy.

However, most people in the modern world follow monotheistic religions (belief in only one God). Judaism, Christianity, and Islam trace their root to a single ancestor Abraham and all these religions believe that human beings are creation of one God (monotheism). The three largest movements within contemporary Judaism (Orthodox, Conservative and Reform) all agree with key theological precepts such as adherence to Scriptures and the celebration of Judaic traditions such as Passover. However, these movements differ in other aspects of religious practices and Reform Judaism is the most liberal form of these three practices. Although Christianity was developed from the first century Jewish reform movement, but Christianity was centered on Jesus Christ and his teachings. Three major religious belief systems are summarized in Table 1.1.

It is interesting to note that two major religions of the world Christianity and Islam originated in the Middle-East while third major religion Hinduism was originated in India. In addition, Judaism was also originated in the Middle-East while other popular religions such as Buddhism and Jainism originated in Indian sub-continent. These are the major religions practiced today in the world. A chronological history of origins of various religions is summarized in Table 1.2. One may wonder why God favored Middle-East and Indian subcontinent to send his messengers.

The Origin of Prayers and Miracles

Prayer is an integral part of all religions. Human communication in the form of some primitive language probably originated approximately 500,000 years ago which coincided with some primitive form of religious practice such as burial of dead and ancient concept of spirit. Concept of symbol including religious symbols were developed about 30,000 years ago and writing around 3200 BC in Mesopotamia. Words of prayer used by ancient cave men cannot be discovered or confirmed, but with development of language rich in vocabulary, ancient forms of prayers practiced during religious ceremonies have indeed been recorded in the history. One of the most ancient forms of prayers, hymns of Rig-Vedas (ancient Hindu scripture) originated between 1700 and 1100 BC. These prayers are still sung in some Hindu religious ceremonies today. The ritual of prayer of ancient Greeks (eighth to sixth century BC to 600 AD) was to pray on their feet, with their hands up to the sky while they were praising Zeus and the other heavenly gods, but during praying to Hades, the king of the underworld, they would kneel and powerfully hit the ground with their heads. Ancient romans (first century BC) who practiced some form of pagan religion also used prayers as a part of their religious ceremonies.

The word prayer (originated from the Latin word *precari* meaning begging) is an act of putting a request to God or some other type of transcendent entity which a practitioner believes is capable of making a change otherwise not possible by normal laws of nature. Prayer could be intercessory in nature, meaning prayer is conducted for the benefit of another person, for example individual or group prayer for recovery of a very ill patient of the community. Prayer can be a part of religious ceremony for example, a church service, or it could be practiced individually in a private place for example chanting mantras during meditation (see Chapter 6). Prayer may involve the use of words, chanting, song, or complete silence. When language is used for prayer, it is usually religious songs or hymns, but it may also take a form of spontaneous utterance of words by the praying person. The main purpose of prayer is to request divine intervention or to praise God for creation. In Hindu worship, majority of mantras are praises for the deity being worshipped as well as request for favors from the deity in the form of abundance, joy, and prosperity. In Islam, daily prayers (praying five times a day) are an essential obligation of a faithful Muslim and it is one of the five pillars of Islam.

A miracle is an event not explicable by natural or scientific laws because miracles occur when God breaks natural laws to perform a miracle and then restores natural laws. A miracle is proof of divine existence. Miracles performed by Jesus Christ such as exorcism, cure of many individuals from incurable diseases, and natural wonders (such as walking on water) are recorded in gospels.

The Catholic Church recognizes miracles as being works of God, either directly, or through the prayers and intercessions of a specific saint or saints. Vatican maintains well documented reports of miracles required for canonization for which at least two miracles are required (except martyr saints). The records of miracles are carefully constructed to serve the canonical tradition and such documents are a part of the Vatican's secret archive which is a privileged source of social, religious, cultural, and medical history. Historical records demonstrated that in the canonization process from 1200 to 1500 AD, medical men were actively appeared as witnesses and in the second half of thirteenth century many canonization processes included at least one medical man who witnessed or provided expert testimony ruling out the possibility that there was a medical explanation for miraculous cure (see bonus section). The Torah, the religious text of Judaism, describes many miracles related to Moses during his time as a prophet and the Exodus of the Israelites. Parting the Red Sea and facilitating the Plagues of Egypt are among the most famous.

Various Theories of Origin of Religion

In general, theories regarding the origin of religion can be broadly classified under two categories; faith based theories (view of divine revelation) and secular based theories. The essential of faith based theories of religion is that divine revelations by prophets are basis of religions. Therefore, religion represents laws revealed by God which should be obeyed without questioning. Faith helps to cope with the stress and sufferings of life. Faith based religion is also used to treat illnesses. Timmons reported the development of a substantive theory to explain an evangelical Christian faith based recovery from addiction where God is considered as the sponsor.[4] However, there are many other theories that attempt to explain origin of religion from a secular point of view. In addition, neurobiologist and psychiatrists attempt to explain religious experiences from known knowledge of structure and function of the human brain (see Chapter 3).[5]

Max Muller's Theory of Origin of Religion

The German philosopher Max Muller (1823-1900) argued that religion originated out of myths and cults which were based upon personification of natural phenomena. According to Max Muller the personification of the sun, sky, mountains, and rocks was the foundation of the earliest known cults. This was the "physical" stage of religion. The "anthropological" stage was the second stage where original nature worship was transformed into ancestor worship. The third stage of religious development was designated as 'psychological' when ancient man further refined his ideas of the controlling forces of the universe to a nonphysical and nonhuman theistic conception. The major monotheistic traditions were representative of this last stage in religious development and currently practiced religions such as Judaism, Christianity, and Islam are monotheistic religions.

Herbert Spencer's Ghost Theory of Religion

Great philosopher, Herbert Spencer (1820-1903) argued that religion was originated from respect given to ancestors. Therefore, gods were derived from early savage experiences of ghosts who were thought to be heroic ancestors of a particular tribe or group. The Hero God was the earliest deity to be worshiped. Spencer also speculated that Animism was a derivative of a belief that the spirits of dead ancestors could reappear as ghosts choosing certain objects in the nature as their dwelling place. Spencer and his followers substantiated their theory by reference to contemporary primitive traditions and analysis of the Hebrew Scriptures and Greek mythology. According to Spencer, man's first reaction to the experience of ghosts was fear. Therefore fear was the fundamental cause of all religious beliefs.

E.B. Taylor and Animistic Theory of Religion

Animism (from Latin word *animus* meaning soul) was the fundamental, supernatural belief system of prehistoric tribes long before emergence of organized religion such as Christianity, Judaism, and Islam. Animism encompassed the belief that there was no separation between the spiritual and physical world because souls or spirits existed, not only in humans, but also in animals, plants, rocks, geographic features such as mountains or rivers, or other entities of the natural environment, including thunder, and wind. Sir Edward Tylor (1832-1917) one of the founders of modern anthropology argued that Animism was the origin of religion where primitive people believed that nature was alive and full of various spirits. Therefore, favor of these spirits and natural forces could be obtained by making offerings to these spirits as well as prying to them. Then Animism and ancestor worship was eventually transformed into first polytheism and eventually into monotheism based religions.

Totemism

Emile Durkheim (1858-1917), a French Sociologist argued that religion originated in totemic rites which were designed to promote the social solidarity of a given tribe. Therefore, religion was needed for socialization of prehistoric humans and symbols of religion (totem) represented realms of supernatural power and strength. The divine laws were in fact laws to maintain harmony and a sense of kinship between individual members of the tribe.

In totemism, each individual in a tribe believed to have a spiritual connection or a kinship with another physical being, such as an animal or plant, often called "spirit-being" or "totem." The word *totem* was derived from the Ojibwa word *ototeman,* meaning "one's brother-sister kin" thus signifying blood relationship between brothers and sisters who had the same mother and who may not marry each other. In English, the word 'totem' was introduced in 1791 by a British merchant and translator who gave it a false meaning in the belief that totem represented guardian spirit which appeared in the form of an animal. However this falsification was due to the fact that the people of Ojibwa tribe wore animal skins and Ojibwa named their clans after those animals that lived in the area and such animals could be considered as either friend or foe. Totemism was traditionally common among indigenous North America tribes (Native American Indians) and parts of South America people in Africa, India, Oceania (especially in Melanesia), Australian Aborigines, African Pygmies, Ugrians, and

West Siberians (hunters and fishermen who also breed reindeer) as well as among tribes of herdsmen in North and Central Asia.

A totem is a spirit being, sacred object, or symbol of a tribe, clan, family, or individual. A totem could be a species of animal, plant, or more rarely a class of inanimate object to which members of clan had very special relationship. Totem did not represent God but something which was highly respected by members of a clan. Totemism can be individual totemism or group totemism. In individual totemism, a person believes that a particular animal or spiritual object may act as his guide throughout his life while in group totemism more than one animals or spiritual objects may be believed to be mystically connected with the entire tribe. Some Native American traditions suggest that each individual is connected with nine different animals that will accompany each person through life, acting as guides. Different animal guides come in and out of one's life depending on the direction that a person is taking and the tasks that should be completed along his/her journey. Though people may identify different animal guides throughout their lifetimes, it is this one totem animal that acts as the main guardian spirit. This Animal Guide offers power and wisdom to the individual when they "communicate" with the animal conveying their respect and trust, but it does not mean that the individual is always associated with the animal because animal guide may not be a pet animal but could be a wild animal such as wolf.

Recently it was reported that a transmission of blood sucking parasites traveled from a python to four humans (two of which died) in a tribes living in Ghana. These particular tribes happen to consider the python their totem animal. Embryonated eggs laid by these parasites are discharged through nasal and fecal mass of pythons and contaminate vegetation and water. In the wild, rodents get infected from this contaminated source and then pythons eat rodents, thus the cycle continues. The individuals infected with the parasite in the report may have been in close contact with a python which was infected with the parasite.[6]

Sigmund Freud's Theory of the Origin of Religion (Psychological Theory)

Sigmund Freud (1856-1939), the founder of psychoanalysis provided theory of psychological origin of religion in his writings; *Totem and Taboo* (1913), *The Future of An Illusion* (1928), *Civilization and its Discontents* (1930) and *Moses and Monotheism* (1939). In Freud's opinion, religion could be considered an expression of underlying psychological neurosis and distress of mankind. In his book *Totem and Taboo,* Freud suggested that in prehistoric times human lived in a patriarchal society where the father had absolute right over all desirable women in the clan. At some point in history, sons rebelled against the father and were expelled from the group by the father (alpha-male). When expelled boys returned to kill their father, whom they both feared and respected, they would distribute females among themselves, but then they felt guilt. Freud argued that the Oedipus complex (where a boy sees his father as a rival to his mother's affection) was also present in prehistoric human society and postulated that all religion was in effect an extended and collective form of guilt and ambivalence to cope with the killing of the father figure (original sin). Therefore, religion is an outshoot of the Oedipus complex, and represents man's helplessness in the world, having to face the ultimate fate of death, the struggle of civilization, and the forces of nature.[7]

In *The Future of An Illusion,* Freud referred religion as an illusion which was perhaps the most important item in the psychical inventory of human civilization. All forms of religious worship and all dogmatic beliefs are our projections of wish with a hope that the God will fulfill our prayers. As a result God is the rationalization of the ideal father and is consequently a purely human creation. In his book *Civilization and its Discontents,* Freud explained that human created religion from an urge to believe in eternity. In his final book, *Moses and Monotheism,* which was published in Freud's year of death, he did not completely abandon his atheist belief but perceived for the first time a value in abstract form of monotheism – worship of an invisible God.[7]

The Terror Management Theory and the Origin of Religion

In social psychology, Terror Management Theory (TMT) deals with the basic conflict of human life. Humans desire to live for eternity, but in reality all humans are mortal. Animals live in the present and do not comprehend mortality but highly evolved humans know that one day death is inevitable. The concept of TMT may be derived from anthropologist Ernest Baker's 1973 Pulitzer Prize-winning *The Denial of Death* where it is argued that all humans are instinctively driven towards survival though at the same time have knowledge of their inevitable mortality.[8] As a result only humans are terrified by fear of death, in which the human body will be destroyed along with the human mind and existence. The terror associated with unstoppable annihilation of human life combined with our desire to live creates a subconscious conflict or anxiety (cognitive dissonance). If life is temporary why does it matter at all? According to Becker, many people spend their entire lives trying to make sense of these conflicting thoughts. We are so afraid of death that we create alternate realities where we will not cease to exist, but rather live on in some other manner and unknown place. According to TMT principles, over time various societies developed "worldviews" that provided protection from fear of annihilation by death. In general "worldview" means a mental image about the world which is a reflection of the moral values of the society including religious values. If individuals become socialized and meet the standards of social behavior and are valued by the society, then they achieve "self-esteem" that facilitates the suppression of fear of death.

Socialization process begins at childhood when children attempt meet the standards set by their parents, such as not fighting with brothers and sisters, attending school, and respecting other family members and neighbors in order to gain approval from their parents. As an adult, individuals obey rules of the society, participate in cultural rituals such as attending religious service according to his/her faith, and develop self-esteem as a good and valuable member of the society. As a result, self-esteem creates an illusion of being protected from death or even transcending death by believing in an afterlife or immortality of soul which is central to most religious beliefs. TMT suggests two different modes of responding to fear of death. One is *"Literal Immortality,"* referring to a non-corporeal (for example soul) aspect of the individual which will live forever after physical death. The other is *"Symbolic Immortality,"* referring to the belief that individuals will live forever through their children (immortality of DNA), or their contribution to the society.[9] For example William Shakespeare is still living through his immortal contribution to literature as well as Isaac Newton and Albert Einstein through their contributions in science.

TMT theory may be compatible with the theory of evolution where anxiety in response to the inevitability of death in prehistoric humans helped them to evolve and eventually live in a society and form moral values. Initially morality was emerged to facilitate peaceful coexistence in a group, but there was still a struggle to deny human mortality. Neanderthals probably buried deceased humans in order to avoid unpleasant odors of dead bodies, but during Upper Paleolithic period (late Stone Age; 40,000–10,000 years ago), burial processes were associated with supernatural beliefs that the dead could achieve eternal life and therefore, food and other necessary things for afterlife were buried along with the deceased. In ancient Egypt a deceased pharaoh was not only buried with food, clothes, and other necessary objects for a meaningful afterlife, but also with his servants so that they could serve him in afterlife. Writings in old pyramids indicate that ancient Egyptians had firm beliefs in afterlife.

In general, all religions of the world guarantee afterlife and eternal existence of soul. Hinduism, Buddhism, and Jainism believe in reincarnation, an assurance of an individual to transcend death through rebirth. Religious beliefs are a powerful means of overcoming the fear of death. It has been documented in psychological research that younger adults tend to express higher levels of death anxiety than older adults and this behavior may be related to increasing levels of religiousness with advancing age. Considering gender, females tend to report greater death anxiety than males. Although some researchers observed lower death anxiety among intrinsic religious persons (religious desire to be closer to God) than extrinsic religious persons (desire to be a part of religious community), such findings have been challenged by other researchers. Moreover, regular attendance to religious service may also reduce death anxiety. As expected, religious doubts increase death anxiety.[10] Krause and Hayward reported lower death anxiety among individuals who felt forgiven by God.[11] However, in a study using 141 older Chinese Buddhist, Hui et al found no correlation between personal belief in reincarnation and death anxiety. The authors commented that not all religious afterlife beliefs have death anxiety buffering power as suggested by TMT perhaps because Buddhists do not view reincarnation as a solace but rather as a renewal of sufferings due to unwholesome karma.[12] Various aspects of religions that alleviate death anxiety are summarized in Table 1.3.

Economic Theories of Religion

There is a long tradition of examining religion within the context of political economy. Karl Marx (1818-1883) famously declared that religion is the opiate of the masses, and explained religion as an epiphenomenon arising from an economic foundation and a mechanism to control labor force. According to Karl Marx, religion represents a sign of the oppressed creature in a hostile world, the heart of a heartless world and the soul of a soulless condition. Max Weber (1864-1920) in his landmark work, *The Protestant Ethic and the Spirit of Capitalism,* argued that religious beliefs were highly influenced by the economic history and religion could act as a force for social changes. Weber wrote that modern capitalism spread quickly, partially due to the worldly ascetic morale of Protestants. Somewhat differing from Marx, Weber dealt with status groups, not with class. In status groups, the primary motivation was prestige and social cohesion. Weber further noticed that in China around 1920, Confucianism was helping the educated elite to maintain access to prestige and power.[13]

More recently, economists have used rational choice theory to explain various aspects of religiosity where they see religions as systems of "compensators" (which compensate for failed goals in material life), and view human beings as rational actors. Therefore, religion can be considered a system of compensation that relies on the supernatural as well as belief in afterlife where life will be wonderful, far exceeding material life standards. In all religious concepts, heaven is a place which is incredibly beautiful with no sufferings or pain. McCullough et al. showed that varieties of religious developments in adulthood are consistent with rational choice theory of religion.[14]

Most religions start as a cult or sect, where a group of people have views and beliefs contrary to social norms. Therefore, this group of people faces high tension with the society. Over time, they tend to either die out, or become more established, thus facing less tension with the society. Cults are new groups with a new novel theology, while sects are attempts to return to mainstream religions to their original purity. There are four models of cult formation: the Psychopathological Model, the Entrepreneurial Model, the Social Model, and the Normal Revelations model.[15] In Psychopathological Model, a religion was founded during a period of severe stress in the life of the founder and foundation of the religion resulted in resolution of the stress. In the Entrepreneurial model, founders of religions acted like entrepreneurs, developing new products (religions) to sell to consumers (to convert people to). Such founders of new religions already had experience in several religious groups before they initiated their own as they took ideas from the pre-existing religions in order to improving the existing religion. In the Social Model of religions it was assumed that religions were founded by means of social implosions. Members of the religious group spent most time with members of the same group and very little time outside the group. The level of affection and emotional bonding between members of a group increased, and their emotional bonds to members outside the group diminished. According to the Social Model, when a social implosion occurred, the group would naturally develop a new theology and rituals to accompany it. According to Normal Revelations Model, a religion was founded when the founder interpreted ordinary natural phenomena as supernatural; for instance, ascribing his or her own creativity in inventing the religion to that of the deity. Some religions are better described by one model than another, though all apply to differing degrees to all religions.

The Theory of Religious Economy views different religious organizations competing for followers in a religious economy, similar to how businesses compete for consumers in a commercial economy. Theorists assert that a true religious economy is the result of religious pluralism, giving the population a wider variety of choices in religion.[16]

The Economic Game Theory, Supernatural Punishment, and Religion

Game Theory was developed by John von Neumann and Oskar Morgenstern. They studied "zero-sum game" where the interests of two players are strictly opposed, in other words: one person's gain should be the other person's loss. Game Theory employs games of strategy representing a situation where two or more participants are faced with choices of action, by which each may gain or lose. The final outcome of a game, therefore, is determined jointly by the strategies chosen by all participants. These are also situations of uncertainty because no participant knows for sure what the other participants are going to decide. Two-person zero-sum games are used by military-strategists. Many-person games are used in the study of economic behavior (Economic Game Theory).

More recently, principles of Game Theory have been applied to study biological evolution and religious behaviors. In one study from the University of British Columbia, fifty volunteers were asked to ration out there money between themselves and the other subjects. Of the thirty-four females and sixteen males, half of the subjects were primed with a God concept prior to participation. When a subject was chosen as a giver subject, he/she could take as many as coins as desired (total ten dollars) knowing that whatever was left would be given to the other subject. Subjects who were not primed for God left on average $1.84 for the other subject but subjects who were primed for God before participation in the game left on average $4.22 for the other subject. The authors concluded that priming with a God concept increased prosocial behavior in an anonymous, economic game and made participants less selfish.[17]

Sanctions imposed on norm violators at the punisher's own expense have powerful cooperation enhancing effects in experimental game situations as well as in real life where violation of laws results in punishment by law enforcement authority. This has been demonstrated using the Game Theory Model when players are provided with certain amount of money and have to decide how much should go to a common accounts (such as public good) and how much to keep in their own private account. With time, as a game unfolds, players contribute lesser amounts of money in the common account. However, if players are given a chance to use targeted punishment against each other the game could unfold differently. When punishment (sanction) is imposed against non-contributors who enjoy free ride, they contribute more to the common account and there is a higher level of cooperation between players. Therefore, punishment is a strong motivating force to modify behavior of a selfish person to make him or her less selfish.[18] Extending this concept, it has been shown that fear of supernatural punishment is a strong motivating force that encourages prosocial behavior.

There has been much speculation why emergence of religious iconography coincided with rapid increases in population densities. Theorists point out that religion's socially cohesive effects are due to collective participations in costly religious rituals and following dietary or other restrictions imposed by the religion. A stranger's faith in some god may serve as an initial reliable cooperative signal but at the same time religious belief could be easily faked. However, religious rituals are often physically taxing and frequently require time commitment which could be otherwise used for some fun activities. Therefore, a stranger faking religious faith initially to be accepted by a group may later not participate in time consuming rituals and could be identified as a "free rider."

However, for individuals with genuine faith in the religion, such rituals must provide some significant reward so that they are willing to participate and follow dietary and other restrictions imposed by the religion. Religion is a cultural variant that confers a selective advantage to an individual as the person is accepted as a valuable member of the group. In general, more demanding religious groups tend to have more committed members.[19]

Religion has a dramatic impact on the development of large scale human societies by encouraging genetically unrelated individuals to cooperate with each other. Religion facilitates acts that benefit others at a personal cost; an example is charitable contributions. If religions are centered on the concept of a God and morality, it is expected that religious people should show stronger altruistic tendencies than non-believers. It has been shown that individuals who pray more often and attend religious services show more prosocial behavior such as charitable donations and volunteerism. Attitudinal surveys also show that religious individuals are perceived to be more trustworthy and more cooperative.[20]

Human societies are based on large scale cooperation between genetically unrelated individuals and such cooperations are based on cultural norms and moral issues of fairness. Humans also reward others who behave fairly and impose sanctions on those who do not behave fairly. One potential means of implementing fairness norms is through culturally postulated supernatural agents such as God. People who believe that a supernatural agent (or God) is policing behavior of all people and will inflict severe punishment to individuals who behave unfairly, out of fear behave according to social norms. Threat of supernatural punishment can suppress selfishness and promote cooperation between members of a society. Religious prime activates the notion that one's behavior is watched by a supernatural agent and under such circumstances primed individuals punish individuals with unfair behavior in order to keep their good standing with a supernatural agent.[21] Religious priming influences an individual to believe that a supernatural agent is watching the person and such belief, although materially fictitious, influences the person in a positive way making him/her more generous to others including strangers.

Sacrifices, Prayers, and Religion

In 1871, Sir E.B. Tylor proposed his theory that sacrifices were gifts to gods to secure their favor or to minimize their hostility. However, in this case one may ask why sacrificial offerings are eaten partly or wholly by worshippers. William Smith hypothesized that the motive of sacrifice was to enhance communion among members of the group as well as between the group and their god. A sacrificial meal was a symbol of communion. In ancient practice of totemism, although an animal was considered a totem and therefore intimately associated with the clan, on sacred days that animal was eaten as a part of sacramental meal that ushered unity between the clan and the totem. It was believed that such ritual should enhance wellbeing of the clan. Ancient Romans practiced animal sacrifice along with prayer in their religious ceremonies.[22]

Chanting prayers during sacrifice is a common element of the practice and dates back to ancient times. Yajur-Veda served as a guidebook to priests who performed Hindu religious ceremonies including sacrifices. In some Hindu rituals, priests perform homa which is worship of sacrificial fire. Sacrifices may be fruits or vegetables or animal sacrifices and one integral part of sacrificial ceremony is chanting Sanskrit prayers. The Hebrew word for sacrifice is *Korban,* meaning "to be brought near." In ancient practices of Judaism, animal sacrifices were practiced with a hope to be nearer to God but with the destruction of the second Temple in 70 AD, practice of animal sacrifice ended in Judaism. At that time ancient rabbis substituted prayer for sacrifice. Nonetheless, the Book of Leviticus (the code book for animal sacrifice) still remained.

The most disturbing aspect of religious sacrifice was human sacrifice. Human sacrifice in the period of the Iron Age was most evident in Denmark, Germany, and Holland. During the Roman Empire, Julius Caesar and other Romans were appalled by the custom of human sacrifice among the Celts, but gladiatorial games and feeding people to lions were regular sport. Human sacrifice was practiced at least five thousand years ago among the early agricultural societies of Europe. Sometimes women were sacrificed to improve the fertility of the land. The ancient civilizations in South America also practiced human sacrifices. Aztec priests believed that the human sacrifices of cutting out beating hearts on top of their pyramids was necessary to keep the sun on its daily path. Ancient Incas sacrificed children and teenagers to the Sun God. Human sacrifice is an example of the dark side that religious superstitions can have.

Conclusion

Religion has many positive effects on human life such as making a person compassionate, prosocial, and enhancing good moral character. However, in order to live peacefully in a society where different members may practice different religions, religious tolerance and cultivation of secular values must be achieved. There is a dark side of religion which is in the form of superstitions and fundamentalism. Common sense tells us if there is a higher being or a creator there must be one creator. Therefore, different religions may prescribe different paths of worship, but all paths eventually lead to the same God. Saint Ramakrishna of nineteenth century India (1836-1886) practiced several religions including Hinduism, Islam, and Christianity, and taught that in spite of differences, all religions are valid and true and they lead to the same ultimate God. Therefore, any religion if followed properly should help us to reunite with the supreme God. Because of different upbringing we may like a particular practice of religion but eventually there is only one God.

Table 1.1 Three major religious belief systems

Religious belief system	Comments	Examples
Polytheism	Belief in many gods and goddesses (includes all ancient religions of the Bronze, Iron, and Axial ages); polytheism later developed into henotheism, where people believed in many gods and goddesses but worship may be directed toward one god or goddess	Many ancient Egyptian, Semitic, Greek, Roman, and Celtic religions were polytheistic. Hindu religion can be considered a polytheistic religion. Ancient religion of Japan "Shinto" is still practiced today. Wicca (pagan) practice is also polytheistic in nature.
Pantheism	Belief that everything in this world/universe is divine (pan means one and theos means god)	A primary example is Taoism. Many new age religions are based on pantheistic philosophy. Spinoza's God is also based on pantheistic philosophy.
Monotheism	Belief in only one God (most of the world population today believes in monotheistic religions)	**Judaism, Christianity, Islam**

Table 1.2 A chronological history of origins of various religions

Time Frame	Comments
Approximately 500,000 -300,000 years ago	Archeological evidence indicating burial of humans; this may be first evidence of origin of religion
Approximately 37,000 -27,000 years ago	Based on archaeological evidence, the Aurignacian culture existed in prehistoric Europe and southwest Asia. The name originates from the type site of Aurignac in the Haute-Garonne area of France. The oldest known example of figurative art, the *Venus of Hohle Fels*, comes from this culture (discovered in September 2008 in a cave at Schelklingen in Baden-Württemberg in southern Germany). This figurine could represent an ancient deity, but it has not been established.
Approximately 30,000 years ago	The Tsodilo Hills in Botswana showed evidence of ancient cave paintings and possibility of place for worship.

Table 1.2 cont.

Time Frame	Comments
Approximately 6600 BC	In Çatalhöyük, Central Anatolia, Turkey, evidence of ancient civilization was discovered. Many female figurines were discovered and could represent goddesses.
Approximately 3300-1300 BC	The Indus Valley Civilization (also known as Harappan civilization) in the northwestern region of the Indian subcontinent (now Pakistan) built its cities of brick, had a roadside drainage system, multistoried houses, and many figurines which could be linked to pre-Vedic religions.
Approximately 2000 BC	Time of Abraham and birth of Judaism
Approximately 2000 -1500 BC	Birth of Hindu religion
1000 BC	Zoroastrianism, founded by Zarathustra and Persia
563 BC	Gautama Buddha, the founder of Buddhism, was born

Table 1.2 cont.

Time Frame	Comments
551 BC	Confucius, the founder of Confucianism, was born.
Approximately fifth century BC	Lao Tzu, a Chinese philosopher, founded Taoism.
599-527 BC	Jainism is an Indian religion which was influenced by twenty-four spiritual leaders (Tirthankaras) where Mahavira (599-527 BC), a contemporary of Gautama Buddha, is considered as the founder of Jainism.
approx. 2 BC–32 AD	Jesus Christ, the Messiah. His followers started Christianity.
570-632 AD	Muhammad founded Islam and the Holy Quran was written based on his revelation.

Table 1.3 Death anxiety and religious belief

- In general, younger people suffer from higher death anxiety than older people due to increasing levels of religiousness with advancing age.
- In general females tend to have greater death anxiety than males.
- Self-identified born again Christian high school students in rural south showed lower death anxiety than who did not identify themselves as born-again Christians.
- Some studies indicated that intrinsic religious people experienced lesser death anxiety than extrinsic religious people, but such findings have been challenged.
- Religious doubts tend to increase death anxiety
- Greater belief in afterlife reduces death anxiety
- Belief that God has forgiven an individual reduces death anxiety
- Non-religious spirituality is not associated with lower death anxiety

Chapter 2
The Origin of Yoga and Meditation

Introduction

Today many people practice yoga throughout the world to derive many health benefits (see Chapter 4). In ancient India, the practice of yoga was integrated with meditation and only individuals who were seeking spiritual growth such as saints (Sanskrit: *munis or rishis*) and their disciples practiced the two. People who practiced yoga in ancient India were also called "yogis" in Sanskrit and this word is still used in India to refer holy men who are seeking union with divinity because yoga and meditation are still integral parts of Hindu spiritual practice (Sanskrit: *sadhana*). Most saints preferred solitary life, living in forests and caves of mountains away from civilization, although some saints were also teachers (Sanskrit: *guru*) who lived with their disciples not far from civilization. Although some saints in ancient India practiced celibacy, some gurus were married and had children. In today's India, there are many saints who prefer to live in isolation at the foothills of the Himalayan Mountains. However, some saints live in hermitages (Sanskrit: *ashram*) with other saints and such *ashrams* may be in a city or near a city.

The word "yoga" is derived from a Sanskrit work "yuj" meaning "union." This union may be the union of body and mind or may transcend beyond body and mind and a yogi may be united with the universe (divinity, God). Yoga which originated in India almost five thousand years ago should not be viewed simply as an ancient exercise protocol because principles of yoga are metaphysical in nature. Yoga is a mind-body integration technique for spiritual advancement. In ancient India yoga and meditation walked hand in hand. Eliade in his book *Yoga, Immortality, and Freedom* defined yoga as, "a collection of specific techniques to seek a truth hidden in the silence and in the inner calm of a people, a fundamental truth which enables one to free the soul from false reality…" .[1]

Although various postures of yoga (asana) can be considered as exercise protocol, Swami Vivekananda (1863-1902) who introduced Vedanta and yoga in the West initially through his famous speech in the Parliament of the World's Religion in Chicago in 1893, commented that the goal of asana in yoga is to learn how to sit still and to keep the body firm so that a practitioner can focus on the mind. A well-known asana known as lotus position (Sanskrit: *padma-asana*) is also a desirable posture to practice meditation

Yoga can be practiced as postures only or in combination with posture (asana) and breathing exercise (pranayama). Although yoga is a non-denominational practice where belief in Hinduism is not a prerequisite, sometimes mantras are repeated during yoga. Meditation was also originated in ancient India and the Sanskrit word for meditation is "*dhyana*." Meditation is a very relaxed, but at the same time, a very alert state of mind. Meditation is a mind body healing practice where a meditator trains his/her mind to suspend the normal stream of various thoughts that typically distract and occupy one's mind. Meditation can be practiced alone or in combination with yoga to achieve many physical and mental health benefits. The primary goal of meditation from ancient time of Vedic, Buddhist, and Taoist practice is to achieve *Samadhi*, a wakeful but tranquil state of total bliss also known as "pure awareness" or "enlightenment." At that state a practitioner is connected with the divine and breaks away from the cycle of birth and death. However, such highest state of mind is not reachable for most of us. Physical and mental health benefits of meditation along with current practice of meditation are discussed in detail in Chapter 5. This chapter focuses on the history of yoga and meditation. Because the initial practice of yoga is connected with Hinduism, a brief description of origin of Hinduism is a necessary predecessor.

Origin of Hinduism

Hinduism is the oldest known religion in the world with approximately one billion followers. Hinduism is also the third most popular religion after Christianity and Islam. The earliest form of Hinduism existed most likely around 3000 BC, but Vedas, the original scriptures of Hinduism, originated much later. The name "Hindu" was derived from the Indus River which currently flows through Pakistan and Northern India. The ancient name of this river was "*Sindhu*" in Sanskrit but Persians pronounced "*Sindhu*" as "Hindu," and the people who lived in Indus Valley became Hindu. Hindu is not a Sanskrit word. The word "India" came from Greeks, when Alexander invaded India, the Macedonian army called river "*Sindhu*" as "Indos" and the land east of the "*Sindhu*" river as "India." It is believed that people who lived in the ancient Indus Valley were Aryans. Originally "Aryans" referred to people who spoke "Indo-European" language; they were typically fair skinned and settled in Northern parts of Iran, Afghanistan, and India (the northwestern part of India where Aryans lived is now Pakistan).[2]

Archeological evidences indicate that there was an ancient civilization in the Indus valley which was called "Harappan" civilization based on the name of the major city Harappa. Unfortunately the ancient writings from that civilization had not been deciphered indicating that they were not related to Sanskrit. The civilization probably dated back to 7000 BC but it was mostly populated around 2300-2000 BC. It has been speculated that the civilization declined due to flooding as well as an invasion of the Aryans. The original language of Harrapan civilization and culture was subdued by invading Aryans. However, Aryan invasion theory is challenged by many scholars and it may be possible that ancient people who lived in different parts of the world including Europe, Mediterranean, Central Asia, Afghanistan, and Northwestern parts of India were actually Aryans. Therefore, Aryans were a heterogeneous group of people who worshipped gods and goddesses. Interestingly, ceremonial fire was an integral part of religious rituals of Aryans. However, before the era of Vedas, archeological evidence in Harappa showed statues engraved on stones that resembled yogi-like figures although, whether such figures indicated some yoga-like practice prior to Vedic period is debatable.

Major Holy Texts in Hinduism and Yoga

In contrast to Christianity and Islam, there is no single Holy Text like the Quran or the Bible in Hinduism.

Four Vedas (in Sanskrit Veda means *knowledge*) are considered as the most ancient scriptures of Hinduism. Another name of Vedas is *sutri* (Sanskrit word meaning *what is heard*). Orthodox Hindus believe that Vedas were not written by humans but Vedic Mantras (hymns) were divinely revealed to Indian saints (Sanskrit: *rishis or munis*). Therefore, Vedas are considered *apaurashaya* (in Sanskrit it means *not created by humans*). Vedas, which were transmitted orally from teacher to disciples, consisted of hymns, charms, spells, and ritual observations but much of such teachings were lost in time and today's versions of Vedas may differ significantly from original versions. Vedas originated between 1700 BC and 800 BC and there are four major ones; the Rig-Veda, the Sama-Veda, the Yajur-Veda, and the Atharva-Veda.

Rig-Veda originated approximately between 1700–1100 BC (Bronze Age) and some verses from Rig-Veda are still recited in Hindu religious ceremonies. Some of the mantras (hymns) found in Rig-Veda are still chanted today during meditation. The Rig-Veda is full of mythological and poetical accounts of the origin of the world, hymns praising various gods and goddesses, as well as prayers for prosperity, wealth, and happiness. The modern version of Rig-Veda contains 1017 hymns because some hymns were lost in time. Most hymns in the Sama-Veda, were borrowed from Rig-Veda. Yajur-Veda served as a guidebook to priests who performed Hindu religious ceremonies including sacrifices during Vedic period. Some scholars opinioned that Yajur-Vedas originated after Rig-Veda but before Sama-Veda. The Atharva-Veda is different from other Vedas because Atharva-Veda contains accounts of magic and healing traditions that have similarity with other Indo-European literature. It was also the last of all Vedas that originated in ancient India.

The religious practices in the Vedic age rested on a priest who performed various rites that often involved animal sacrifices. *Homa* (Sanskrit word meaning ceremonial fire) was an integral part of *Yagna* (Sanskrit word for Hindu religious ritual) where offerings were made to God. Although the practice of yoga was mentioned in Vedas, in the late Vedic period known as Upanishadic or Vedantic period, practice of yoga and meditation became more integrated in the spiritual practice of Hinduism. The Upanishads are a continuation of the Vedic philosophy, and were composed between 800 BC and 400 BC. There are more than two hundred Upanishads but Brhadaranyaka and the Chandogya were the two earliest Upanishads composed probably between the seventh and sixth centuries BC, before birth of Gautama Buddha, the founder of Buddhism. The three other early composed Upanishads: Taittiriya, Aitareya, and Kausitaki were probably also pre-Buddhist in origin, composed between the sixth and fifth centuries BC. There were many references of yoga in various Upanishads because during that period Hindus were deviating from elaborate rituals of *Yagans* and focusing on the practice of yoga and meditation in order to connect with the divine. Upanishads elaborated practical ways on how the soul (Sanskrit: *Atman*) can be united with the supreme God (*Brahman*) through meditation and good deeds (Sanskrit: *karma*). In the later part of this period Sanskrit epics (Ramayana and Mahabharata), and Puranas (Sanskrit word meaning ancient) were composed. However, Upanishads represent the core of Hindu philosophy.

One of the founding religious texts of Hinduism is the Bhagavad Gita meaning "Songs of the God." It was written between 300 and 200 BC and focused on how the human soul can be united with the divine through yoga and good deeds. The Bhagavad Gita consists of eighteen chapters, seven hundred verses described in the form of a conversation between Krishna and Arjuna on the battlefield of Kurukshetra (epic battle described in Mahabharata) prior to the start of the Holy War (Sanskrit: *Dharma Yudha*). Arjuna was reluctant to participate in the war because he did not want to kill his cousins who were the opponents. At that point Krishna, the charioteer explained to Arjuna his duties as a warrior and educated Arjuna on Vedantic philosophies and also revealed his true identity as an incarnation of Lord Vishnu. After realizing Krishna's true form, Arjuna agreed to fight and finally his side (Pandavas) won the battle.

Major teaching of Gita is that soul is immortal and every human should be engaged in good karma (daily actions of life) without expectation of any favorable result (Sanskrit word: *nishkam karma* meaning *selfless action*). An example *of nishkam karma* is to work very hard without expecting any salary increase or even praises from the boss. In Bhagavad Gita, Krishna also explained three different approaches to break the cycle of birth and death with an ultimate goal of God realization. These three practices include complete devotion to God (Sanskrit: *bhakti-yoga*), selfless and desire-less action (niskam karma or *karma-yoga*) and path of knowledge to comprehend the true nature of God (Sanskrit: *Jnana-yoga*). Krishna did not disrespect the physical world but advised everyone to live in harmony with divine laws. Although Bhagavad Gita described importance of yoga for spiritual growth, the major ancient text on yoga was "Yoga Sutra" wrote by saint Patanjali. This book is still considered as the authentic book of yoga and many yoga teachers still read this book as the reference book on yoga. Mention of yoga in major Holy Hindu texts is summarized in Table 2.1.

Practice of Yoga and Meditation in the Vedic Age and Post Vedic Age

In ancient Vedic time, saints who were actively involved in elaborate Hindu religious ceremonies (Yagna) were also yogis because they practiced yoga and meditation so that they could calm their minds in order to focus on rituals and correctly pronouncing Vedic mantras. Great emphasis was placed on correctly chanting Vedic mantras because if not pronounced properly gods or goddesses may become upset. Moreover, those rituals were very time consuming and proper postures (asana) were very important for saints who performed such rituals. Moreover, these saints also must achieve mastery in proper yogic breathing (pranayama) because ancient practice of yoga also placed great emphasis on respiration as well as respiratory control because the way a person breathed was considered important for spiritual growth. According to Taittiriya Upanishad, there are five levels of existence and for optimal health and emotional well-being there must be a balance between these states of existence:

- Existence in physical level
- Existence in subtle energy level (Sanskrit: *prana*)
- Existence in the mental level based on instinct
- Existence in the mental plane based on intellect
- Existence in the optimal state of health and emotional well-being.[3]

The most common imbalance in the level of subtle energy could be manifested by erratic breathing due to mental anguish as well as nervousness. A yogi must correct irregular breathing. Moreover, getting rid of mental anguish and nervousness is essential to make spiritual progress. This is the reason why proper breathing was so much emphasized in ancient texts related to the practice of yoga. Another ancient yoga text, *Hatha Yoga Pradipika* written around 300 AD, also mentioned the importance of proper breathing during yoga.[4]

In the ancient Vedic period (1700 BC–500 BC), religious rituals (*Yagna*) were an integral part of the practice of Hinduism, but due to enormous cost, only kings and very wealthy people were able to conduct such rituals. However, in the post Vedic period (500–200 BC), Buddhism and Jainism evolved in India as major religions had offered alternative pathways for spiritual growth. At that period expensive *Yagnas* lost their glory and common people were more focused on individual worship, yoga, and meditation for spiritual growth. In sharp contrast to *Yagnas,* where many animals were sacrificed, both Buddhism and Jainism preached non-violence to all living creatures and killing animals even for food is strictly prohibited in both religions. Therefore, followers of Jainism even today in India and elsewhere are strict vegetarians and many Buddhist are also vegetarians. Although ancient Hindus ate meat, some Hindus today are also vegetarian. Some scholars think that this is due to influence of Jainism.

Yoga and meditation are also incorporated in spiritual practice of both Buddhism and Jainism. Siddhartha Gautama (Buddha; 563 BC–483 BC) who was the founder of Buddhist religion was born approximately 2500 years ago in Lumbini, Nepal as a son of Shuddhodhana, the King of Kapilavastu and his Queen Maya Devi. He left the royal palace at the age of twenty-nine to seek enlightenment and experiment with various methods of meditation, mind control, breathing techniques (pranayama), and sensory withdrawal. However, the ultimate stage of enlightenment was still unattainable. Finally he practiced extreme fasting and almost died. Realizing he was near death but did not achieve his goal, he decided to give up fasting. At that time a passerby woman Sujata offered him a bowl of rice pudding containing milk, rice, and sugar (see Chapter 3). After eating rice pudding Siddhartha sat again under the Bodhi tree to meditate and effortlessly achieved his desired enlightenment. Although Buddha strongly discouraged his disciples from worshiping him or his image, after his death numerous statues of Buddha were constructed and in many of these statues, Buddha was sitting in the "lotus position," an asana described in ancient Indian texts.

Jainism was preached by Mahavira (599 BC–527 BC) when Buddhism was popular in India. It is important to mention that both Buddhism and Jainism are practiced today by many followers. Meditation is a central practice in Jainism to attain spiritual growth. The goal of meditation in Jainism is self-realization and to achieve a high state of consciousness that is beyond any material attachment. At that state an individual (jiva) can truly see his or her soul (atma). Meditation is also important in Buddhism, but unlike in Hinduism or Jainism, Buddha did not talk about existence of the human soul or God. Therefore, Buddhism can be considered an atheist religion although later followers of Buddha (Mahayana) believed in concepts of gods and goddesses similar to Hinduism. In fact some of the goddesses worshipped today in India originated from goddesses worshipped by Mahayana

Buddhists. Buddha believed in rebirth but not transmigration of the human soul from a dead body to a new living body. Buddha preached that the cause of rebirth is attachment of a human being with life. When a person is completely detached from this world mentally or emotional there should be no rebirth as the person will achieve "Nirvana." Nirvana is not like going to heaven but rather a state of "non-existence."

Patanjali's Yoga Sutra

Patanjali wrote the famous *Yoga-Sutra* book which is still considered as the classical ancient text on yoga. The book was probably written around 200 AD, although some scholars opine that the book maybe written as late as 400 AD Swami Vivekananda wrote a comprehensive book on the Yoga-Sutra of Patanjali in English. After that there are several excellent English translations of Yoga-Sutra of Patanjali which are currently available in the U.S. market. According to Yoga-Sutra (Sutra in Sanskrit means *thread that binds all sutras together to a complete text*), the most auspicious time to meditate is between four in the morning and six in the morning. This timeframe is called "Brahmamuhutra." A well-known quote from Swami Satchidananda's book related to Yoga-Sutra is:

> "We are not going to change the whole world, but we can change ourselves and feel free as bird. We can be serene even in the midst of calamities and by our serenity, make others more tranquil. Serenity is contagious. If we smile at someone, he or she will smile back. And a smile costs nothing. We should plague everyone with joy. If we are to die in a minute why not die happily, laughing?"[5]

The Yoga-Sutra of Patanjali has 196 sutras (verses) and the book is divided into four parts (Table 2.2). Although yoga was emphasized in the Holy Text of Bhagavad Gita, sage Patanjali made the first effort to compile several practices of yoga and their effects systematically in one book. His Sutras suggest that yoga practice helps to reach a state of mental calm which is synonymous with mental equilibrium described in Bhagavad Gita. Yoga Sutra provides a manual of physical practices (postures; asana) and breathing exercises (pranayama) by which one gradually progresses towards a mental calm state and later by meditation can ultimately achieve further spiritual progress. The first part of the book focused on how to achieve "*yoga-chitta-vritti-nirodha*" a Sanskrit word meaning stopping fluctuations or wandering nature of mind. It can also be interpreted as blocking all illusions or misconceptions from human consciousness and when a yogi achieves mastery in this practice then he/she can progress towards "Samadhi," the enlightened state of consciousness. Therefore, yoga can be also viewed as a method of restraining activities of the mind so that mind can stay calm and stop wandering. In the second part of the book, Patanjali described the practice of yoga, detailing various postures (asana) and also obstacles to yoga practice. Also in the second part of the book he described famous Astanga yoga (eight limb yoga) and action yoga (*kriya* yoga). In the third part, Patanjali discussed various supernatural powers (Sanskrit: *Siddhi*) a yogi may achieve through practice of yoga. In the fourth part of the book the authors discussed how to achieve complete liberation by uniting with the supreme God (moksha). Unlike Buddha, Patanjai believed in a supreme God (Sanskrit: *Ishvara*).

Astanga or eight-limb yoga described by Patanjali is probably the most comprehensive manual of yoga practice. These eight limbs of yoga are summarized in Table 2.3. Patanjali's eight-limb yoga and underlying philosophy described in the Yoga-Sutra came to be called "Raja-yoga which is the basis of all modern yoga practices.[6] Following sage Patanjali's description of eight-limb yoga to achieve Samadhi or total liberation (enlightenment), Swami Vivekananda (1863-1902) who first introduced Hinduism and principles of yoga in the West, expanded the concept of yoga to incorporate yoga in everyday life. He conceptualized four ways of practicing yoga as a part of modern day life that was consistence with the concept of Astanga yoga described first by Patanjali. These four steps include:[7]

Performing work (duties) with a selfless attitude (Karma-yoga)

- Acquiring an in-depth knowledge about spirituality (Jnana yoga)
- Devotion to God (Bhakti yoga)
- Practice yoga for spiritual growth (Raja Yoga)

Raja (royal) yoga described by Swami Vivekananda is based on principles of Yoga Sutra. Beginning in the twentieth century, yoga became more widely practiced in the West. After Swami Vivekananda, many masters introduced various forms of yoga; for example, Iyenger yoga introduced by B.K.S Iyenger, Kriya yoga by Pramahamsa Yogananda, Bikram yoga by Bikram Choudhury, etc. (see Chapter 4). Various, voluntarily regulated yoga breathing techniques (pranayama) have different effects on the human metabolism. During high frequency yoga breathing (Sanskrit: *kapalabhati*) energy is derived from carbohydrate but after such practice energy is derived from fats. Meditation practices also have distinctive effects on the endocrine system, autonomic system, nervous system, brain areas attention, executive function, and emotion regulation (see Chapter 5).[8]

Hatha Yoga Pradipika

Hatha Yoga Pradipika (light on hatha yoga) was written by Swami Svatamarama, a disciple of Swami Gorakshanath in the fifteenth century. It is a classical text on hatha yoga. This book simplified Patanjali's Yoga-Sutra by eliminating the first two limbs of yoga (ethical rules and self-purification). Instead it focused on the physical purity of the body and good moral conduct. The ultimate purpose of Hatha Yoga is to awaken Kundalini energy present at the base of the spine and to advance Kundalini energy to the crown chakra, ultimately to achieve a blissful state of mind known as samadhi.[9]

Conclusion

This chapter provides a brief historical overview of origin of yoga and meditation. An in-depth discussion on books such as Yoga Sutra or Hatha Yoga Pradipika is beyond the scope of the book. For learning yoga this author recommends attending a yoga school or to find a qualified yoga instructor. Although the goal of yoga and meditation is to achieve enlightenment, yoga can be practiced for the many health benefits it provides. Meditation can be practiced for mental calmness in addition to the physical and mental health benefits. You do not have to be a Hindu to practice yoga and/or meditation.

Table 2.1 Yoga and major Holy Texts of Hinduism

Holy text of Hinduism	Approximate time frame	Comments
Vedas: Rig-Veda, Sama-Veda, Yajur-Veda and the Atharva-Veda	1700 BC to 800 BC	Vedas were transmitted orally from masters to students and as a result many original verses have been lost or altered. Yoga was mentioned in the Vedas because during holy ceremonies (*Yagna*) saints had to sit in various positions (*asana*) and concentrate on properly reciting verses (*mantras*).
Upanishads	800 BC to 400 BC	There are more than two hundred Upanishads which focused on interpretation of the knowledge of the Vedas. Yoga and meditation were addressed in several Upanishads as a spiritual practice at a time in India when there was a shift from very expensive religious ceremonies (*Yagna*) to individual spiritual practice through yoga and meditation. Upanishads described in detail the spiritual path which a man should follow in order to reunite the human soul (*atman*) with the supreme God (*Brahman*). Later Buddhism and Jainism were preached in India which also favored meditation for spiritual growth along with non-violence (both Buddhism and Jainism forbid killing animals and vegetarian diet is a must).

Table 2.1 cont.

Holy text of Hinduism	Approximate time frame	Comments
Ramayana	500–400 BC	An epic written by Sage Valmiki is considered a Holy Text because it describes the story of Rama, who was a reincarnation of Lord Vishnu. To my knowledge there is no specific mention of yoga in this epic.
Mahabharata	300–400 BC	Written by Saint Vyasa, Mahabharata is another epic where a war between Pandava and Kaurava Princes takes place at the battlefield of Kurukshetra. It is the longest epic ever written with more than 200,000 verse lines. The teaching of Lord Krishna to Arjuna at the battlefield of Kurukshetra was the basis of another Hindu Holy Text, the Bhagavad Gita.
Bhagavad Gita	300–400 BC	This is a very valuable Holy Text which most Hindus still read today. Gita is a part of the epic of Mahabharata. The Gita mentioned four forms of yoga to break away from the cycle of birth and death to achieve liberation (*moksha*).
Yoga-Sutra by Patanjali	200 AD (or 400 AD)	Written in four parts, this book is the most comprehensive, practical manual of practicing yoga.

Table 2.1 cont.

Holy text of Hinduism	Approximate time frame	Comments
Hatha Yoga-Pradipika	Fifteenth century	This book consists of four chapters and describes eighty-four yoga postures (asana).

Table 2.2 Four parts of Yoga-Sutra by Patanjali

Name of Chapter	Number of verses (*Sutra*)	Comment
Samadhi Pada	51	Samadhi is the blissful state of mind where a yogi is in union with divinity. This is also the enlightened state of mind where all knowledge of the universe is known to the yogi.
Sadhana Pada	55	Sadhana is a Sanskrit word meaning *practice of spirituality*. In this part Patanjali described two forms of yoga: Ashtanga Yoga (eight-limb yoga) and Kriya Yoga (action).
Vibhuti Pada	56	This part also describes the practice of yoga and meditation, but the focus is on the benefits of yoga and what super-natural powers (Vibhuti) may be obtained by a yogi after practicing yoga tradition over time.
Kaivalya Pada	34	Although the Sanskrit word *Kaivalys* means isolation, this part describes how the ultimate goal of yoga practice is breaking away from the cycle of birth and death and achieving liberation (moksha or mukti). It is important to note that "moksha" described in Yoga-Sutra is not conceptually the same as "Nirvana" described in Buddhism.

Table 2.3 Astanga Yoga (eight-limb yoga)

Sanskrit name	English translation	Comment
Yama	Ethical rules of conduct in Hinduism	The five ethical rules listed by Patanjali include non-violence, truthfulness, non-stealing, practicing celibacy (or sexual discipline such as a monogamous relationship), and free from all greed.
Niyama	Self-purification	The five self-purification principles include cleanliness of body, contentment, disciple (perseverance), study of Vedas (scriptures), and devotion to God (*Ishvara*).
Asana	Physical postures	Yoga postures should be held for as long as the practitioner is comfortable.
Pranayama	Voluntary breath regulation	Various techniques of breathing regulation manipulate vital energy of the body. It is believed that vital energy flows through subtle channels (*nadis such as ida and pingala*) through the body.

Sanskrit name	English translation	Comment
Pratyahara	Sense withdrawal	This is a mental exercise to calm one's mind by stopping mind-wandering. This can be done by withdrawing the mind from the external stimuli and turning mind inward.
Dharana	Mind concentration	This step is designed for further calming the mind by practicing mind concentration. This mind control is essential for the next step which is meditation.
Dhyana	Meditation	Meditation is a very relaxed but aware state of mind where the mind is completely withdrawn from any outside stimuli. Meditation yields insight and self-knowledge.
Samadhi	Enlightenment	Enlightenment is the ultimate goal of yoga. It occurs when a yogi is united with the supreme and thus breaks away from the cycle of birth and death. This is the ultimate blissful state when a human is always in contact with the divine.

Chapter 3
Spirituality, Religion, and the Human Brain

Introduction

Primitive religious beliefs originated around 500,000 years ago. This is when humans began burying the dead and practicing some burial rituals. Religion endured this vast span of human history because it provides humans with a powerful coping skill dealing with disappointments and sufferings. Religion makes humans prosocial and provides tools to deal with death anxiety by giving the hope of immortality of the soul or an afterlife. Religion binds together people with common values and beliefs and acts as a fabric of the society even in secular countries.

Freud considered religion as an illusion and observed similarities between religion and obsessional neurosis. Some psychiatrists attempt to describe mystic experiences of saints as symptoms of mental illness.[1] Finding similarities between schizophrenia and religious experience (such as hearing voices) by some psychiatrists also validated such hypothesis. According to *Astonishing Hypothesis* of Frances Crick, all human experiences including joy, sorrow, memories, ambitions, free will, personal identity, and even spiritual experience are in fact no more than behavior of a vast assembly of nerve cells (neurons) and their associated molecules such as neurotransmitters.[2]

Religious Experience

Religion is one of the five major evolutionary, behavioral phenomena of humans (the other four are language, advanced tool making, music and art). The religious experience has both an explicit component (vision, voices, etc.) and a vague, numinous component, which is mainly associated with a strong emotion. Such numinous experiences may include an awareness of the presence of a divine being, experiencing timelessness, feelings of unconditional love, etc. Religious experiences are always perceived by individuals as a real life experience, not a hallucination. Moreover, religious experiences are worldwide phenomenon experienced by people of different religions and cultures. Interestingly, children of atheists may have religious experiences. Therefore, it could be concluded that religious experiences are universal characteristics of human beings. Major religious/spiritual perceptions are as follows:

- Awareness of presence of a divine being
- Moving beyond perception of personal space and time
- Spiritual awe
- Altered state of consciousness
- Feeling oneness with the universe (God)
- Feeling of joy and unconditional love
- Feeling of enlightenment [3]

According to surveys in the U.S., Britain, and Australia, 20–49% of people surveyed reported having religious (numinous) experiences.[4] Genetic studies involving identical and fraternal twin pairs raised apart suggest that genetic factors may account for 50% of interindividual variance in religious interest and attitude [5]. The human brain is very complex and even today there are still unsolved scientific mysteries of the brain. It is possible that through evolutionary pathways the human brain has evolved enough to be wired for a "God realization." Whether the human brain is hardwired to create the concept of God or the human brain is hardwired to perceive God is an ongoing debate in theology and science.

Overview of the Human Brain

The skull protects the human brain from injury and under the skull the human brain is further protected by three strong membranes (meninges) that cover both the brain and the spinal cord. Cerebrospinal fluid (CSF) is a clear, colorless bodily fluid that flows in the space between the two membranes and the spine. Cerebrospinal fluid is produced in the choroid plexus of the brain from blood. The human brain on average weighs approximately 1.4 kilograms or three pounds and has three main components; the cerebrum, the cerebellum, and the brainstem. The cerebrum is the largest and most developmental part of the human brain. The brain stem connects the brain with the spinal cord so that communication can flow between the central nervous system (brain, brain stem, and spinal cord) and the peripheral nervous system (nerves in the remaining parts of the body). Another way to identify major brain areas is to divide the brain into forebrain, midbrain, and hindbrain. Forebrain is the largest area of the brain containing the cerebrum, thalamus, and hypothalamus. The cerebrum also envelops the midbrain as well as the brainstem. The brainstem is the region of the brain that connects the cerebrum with the spinal cord. In addition to the midbrain, the brainstem also contains the medulla oblongata and the pons (in the region of the hindbrain). Motor and sensory neurons travel through the brain stem allowing for the relay of signals between the brain and the spinal cord. The midbrain is the smallest part of the brain located below the cerebrum, joining the diencephalon (thalamus and hypothalamus) with the hindbrain (above pons). Therefore, the midbrain can be viewed as a bridge, joining the forebrain with the hindbrain. The hindbrain is the lower part of the brain, consisting of pons, the medulla oblongata, and the cerebellum (Figure 1).

The cerebrum, the largest part of human brain is divided into two halves (right and left hemispheres). These two halves are joined by the corpus callosum, a collection of nerve fibers. The left hemisphere of the brain controls the muscles of the right side of the body and vice versa. The left hemisphere is associated with language, analytical skills, such as science and math while the right hemisphere is associated with innovation, intuition, art, music, and overall creativity. However, current research indicates that the two sides work together to perform a wide variety of tasks.[6]

Each cerebral hemisphere has four lobes, the frontal, parietal, temporal, and occipital. The outermost layer of the cerebrum is called "cortex" and this part is responsible for cognition, personality, and coordination of complex movements. The cortex has a folded, wrinkled structure giving it a much greater surface area in a limited volume thus accommodating more nerve cells. The cerebral cortex can be classified into two parts, the large area is the neocortex and the much smaller area is the allocortex. Below the cortex lies the white area of the brain that contains nerve fibers. Another region of the brain is the limbic system which is located at the top of the brainstem and consists of amygdala, thalamus, hypothalamus, and hippocampus. The pituitary gland is located close to the hypothalamus and the hypothalamus, along with pituitary glands, secret hormones that are essential for life. The brainstem is located underneath the limbic system. Activities of various parts of the human brain are presented in Table 3.1.

The function of the human brain is due to the presence of one hundred billion nerve cells (neurons). Everything humans do relies on neurons communicating with each other. Moreover, each neuron may be connected to one thousand other neurons thus making over one hundred trillion connections. As a result the human brain is lot more complex than the most advanced computers. The brain can also process information extremely fast, up to three hundred milliseconds.

A nerve cell has three basic parts: a *cell body* containing the nucleus (also DNA), cytoplasm, cell organelles; *dendrites* which branch off the cell body; and axons which send impulses and extends from the cell body to deliver impulses to other neurons. Synapses are small gaps between neurons where messages move from one neuron to another, mostly as chemical signals. When a neuron is activated, a small electrical signal is generated (action potential) and travels very quickly along the axon and then a chemical messenger (neurotransmitter) is released. The neurotransmitter travels through the synapse and binds to the receptor of the receiving neuron's dendrite. Then the entire process may be repeated.

Common neurotransmitters are acetylcholine, serotonin, dopamine, GABA (gamma-aminobutyric acid), epinephrine, nor-epinephrine, and glutamate. Their functions are summarized in Table 3.2. However, more than 180 neurotransmitters have been identified by scientists. Neurotransmitters also can be divided under two broad groups; inhibitory or excitatory. Excitatory neurotransmitters stimulate neurons while inhibitory neurotransmitters have calming effects. Neurotransmitters play important roles in the everyday function of an individual. Deficiency of a neurotransmitter may cause psychiatric illness.

Electroencephalogram (EEG) is a test that records the overall electrical activity of the brain as brain waves (brain waves are bands are electromagnetic waves). For this purpose special sensors (electrodes) are placed over the scalp and these electrodes are hooked by wires to a computer. In general, brain waves represent a collection of electrical impulses generated by billions of neurons during communicating with each other. There are four types of brain waves. Higher frequency beta-waves (12-30 Hertz; or 12-30 cycles per second) are the dominant wave during the normal waking state of a human. The alpha waves (8-12 cycles per second) have a slower frequency than beta-waves and represent a deeply relaxed, but waking state of mind usually with eyes closed. This may occur when a person takes a short break after completion of an assignment. The next, slower frequency brain waves are theta waves (4-8 cycles per second) which are associated with deep relaxation as well as sleep and dream. Theta waves are also associated with increased intuition, emotional connections, and creativity. The slowest waves are known as delta waves (0.5-4 cycles per second) which are associated with deep sleep. More recently neurobiologists pay attention to a high frequency gamma (40-80 cycles per second) waves which are associated with higher mental activity and consolidation of information from all parts of the brain. Some Tibetan monks during meditation show presence of gamma waves in the EEG (see Chapter 5). There are also many applications of EEG analysis including diagnosis of epilepsy, attention deficit disorders, and sleep disorders[7].

The Highly Evolved Human Brain and the Origin of Religion

As mentioned earlier, human brain has one hundred billion neurons and an estimated storage capacity of 1.25 trillion bytes, indicating that cognitive capacity of the human brain is virtually limitless. The brainstem is considered the oldest part of the brain from an evolutionary standpoint. The brainstem controls basic survival needs such as eating, breathing, and response to external stress such as fight of flight. The limbic system of the brain controls emotion but is also involved in memory storage and processing. The cerebral cortex has grown out of the limbic system. In all of human evolution, the latest evolutionary developed part of the brain is the neocortex which is involved in higher functions such as abstract thinking. When humans learn new things, the chemistry of neurons in the neocortex area is altered.[8]

Approximately two million years ago the brain size of ancient humans was 400-600 cubic centimeters and those early humans were able to walk upright. Between two million years and 800,000 years ago both the body size and the brain size of humans were increased, around 800,000 years ago the average human brain size exceeded one thousand cubic centimeters. However, between 800,000 and 200,000 years ago only the brain size of early humans was increased but not the body size. A final leap of increased brain size took place approximately 180,000 years ago when prehistoric humans had a brain size approaching the brain size of modern humans (1200-1400 cubic centimeters).[9] The large human brain may be responsible for the long life span of humans compared to apes. Romantic love and monogamy is attributed to the large brain size. Research has indicated that birds that prefer to live in pairs have a relatively larger brain size compared to body weight. There is some evidence that early humans, around 150,000 years ago, started pair bonding and practicing monogamy. The romantic love among prehistoric human couples played an important role in the evolution of humans.[10]

Robin Dunbar, professor of Anthropology at Oxford University argued that the critical event in the evolution of the neocortex in

Homo sapiens took place approximately 500,000 years ago and such neocortex was large enough to process complex, social phenomenon such as symbolic language and religion. Professor Dunbar also argued in his "Social Brain Hypothesis" that primates and humans have usually larger brains with respect to body size compared to all other vertebrates. Primates and later humans evolved to have a large brain size including the neocortex to manage a complex social system (In primates, the neocortex occupies 50% of the brain, but in humans the neocortex represents 80% of the brain). Socialization of prehistoric humans and the understanding of human mortality could be considered as the origin of religion due to the increased brain size.[11]

In prehistoric time, evolutionary changes that favored larger brains helped Savannah hunters to live in groups and accept the inevitability of human mortality. In order to deal with human mortality, prehistoric humans may have created a belief in an afterlife and a spiritual life and that could be considered as the origin of ancient religion. Early humans also learned empathy, sharing food, restraining selfishness, building a more cooperative group, and eventually establishing a social hierarchy in order to live in a group. In the opinion of psychologist Matt J. Rossano, religion was built upon morality by expanding social scrutiny of individual behavior to include supernatural agents such as dead ancestors, spirits, and eventually God. This was an effective strategy to restrain selfishness of individual members in order to achieve more cooperation between members. Social norms were communally agreed upon, which in part were responsible for unique human forms of cooperation and social organization. Rituals and ritualized behaviors were essential to the transmission and reinforcement of social norms.[12]

Superior pattern processing of the highly evolved human brain is the key to religiosity/spirituality. Superior pattern processing is also a unique feature of the human brain and is responsible for intelligence, development of language, imagination, invention, and emotion. During human evolution, pattern processing capacity became increasingly sophisticated due to the expansion of the cerebral cortex, particularly the pre-frontal cortex, and other brain regions responsible for image processing. However, the highly evolved, superior pattern processing capabilities of the human brain also created imaginary entities such as ghosts and gods.[13] Evolutions of human brain linked to the origin of religion are listed in Table 3.3.

Various Regions of the Brain and Religious Experience

Various regions of the brain have been implicated in religious experiences. Morality is the most sophisticated feature of human judgment and behavior. From a neuroanatomic point of view, morality is a result of large, functional network of the brain including both cortical and subcortical structure. While the prefrontal cortex is involved in making moral decisions, the temporal lobe of the brain is involved in mind control. In addition, the amygdala, hippocampus, and basal ganglia all contribute to making moral decisions. Brain areas that are responsible for making moral decision are influenced by genetic factors as well as environmental factors including religion[14]. Morality and religious beliefs are sometimes interconnected. Wain and Spinella reported that the prefrontal cortex plays an important role in morality, religion, and paranormal beliefs of humans. Hyper-religiosity may be related to hyper-function of the medial prefrontal cortex.[15,12]

The Limbic System and Religious Experience

The limbic system is located at the top of the brainstem and consists of the amygdala, thalamus, hypothalamus, and hippocampus. It is considered the emotional center of the brain. This system plays an important role in the perception of God and religion. There are evidences indicating that prehistoric humans had strong belief in afterlife and transmigration of the soul 100,000 years ago. When humans first perceived the concept of God is difficult to establish but Neanderthals and other Homo saliences were engaged in complex religious rituals approximately between 150,000 and 35,000 BC. Interestingly approximately 32,000 years ago ancient humans started cave painting which included some religious objects. An ancient Tibetan book of death described accounts of those who had undergone near-death experiences where an individual travelled through a dark tunnel and eventually experienced the light of the heaven and were greeted by dead relatives or a being of light.[16] This description is similar to near-death experience reported in recent medical literature and described in several books, some of them written by physicians based on their research or personal experience in the field.

Prehistoric humans (Neanderthal, Cro-Magnon, etc.) buried dead people in a sleeping position with offerings at the grave. This indicates that early humans were able to experience love, fear, religion, and mystical experiences. The human limbic system and temporal lobe have been implicated in fear, love, intense emotion, religious, and spiritual beliefs. The amygdala and inferior temporal lobe appeared to be developed in Neanderthals, Cro-Magnons, and other early humans enabling them to have had religious and spiritual beliefs. More interestingly, the religious symbol of the "cross" was first engraved around 60,000–100,000 years ago. Probably other religious symbols such as spiritual triangles and circles were also perceived by ancient humans approximately 30,000–100,000 years ago. The activation of neurons in the amygdala-temporal lobe were associated with religious feelings. The neurons that are responsible for religion/mystical experiences were evolved by 30,000 years ago or possibly 100,000 years ago. The amygdala is intimately interconnected with the hypothalamus; it enables humans to experience love and spirituality.[17]

Saver and Robin proposed the Limbic-Marker Hypothesis for religious experiences. According to these authors, all human experiences, including religious experiences, are based on brain functions. Most religious experiences such as religious love, fear, and awe are similar to non-religious, emotional experiences such as love, fear, and awe. Therefore, the human limbic system and subcortical networks are responsible for such emotions regardless if induced by religion or not. According to Limbic-Marker Hypothesis of religion, the perceptual and cognitive content of numinous experiences are seen as similar to those of ordinary experiences except that the limbic system tags such ordinary experiences in such a way that such experiences appear as profound and extraordinary.[18]

The Temporal Lobe, Prefrontal Cortex, and Religious Experience

The temporal lobe is another part of the brain implicated in religious experience. Religious experiences are often noticed in patients with temporal lobe epilepsy. Several phenomena linked to altered activity of the limbic system, such as dreams, hallucinations, depersonalizations, near-death experiences, and déjà-vu can be easily interpreted as religious experiences. Based on research using single photon emission computed tomography scan, Newberg et al. speculated that various religious activities such as meditation, prayer, and religious rituals stimulate the limbic system of the brain, thus heightening the activity of hypothalamus, amygdala, and hippocampus. As a result metabolism in the prefrontal cortex of the brain is increased.[19] Schjoedt et al. using functional magnetic resonance imaging technique observed that praying activated a strong response in the temporal region, the medial prefrontal cortex, the temporoparietal junction (where temporal and parietal lobe meet), and the precuneus (a structure in the parietal lobe of the brain, near the juncture between the two hemispheres). Therefore, praying to God or being connected to God is an interpersonal interaction comparable to a normal interpersonal interaction between two people in a social context.[20]

Asp et al. proposed "False Tagging Theory" to explain religious beliefs. According to this theory the process of belief occurs in two stages. In the first stage, all ideas presented are initially believed by an individual. In the second stage of processing information, doubts may arise thus tagging an idea as false. The prefrontal cortex is necessary for false tagging. Any damage to the prefrontal cortex should result in "doubt deficit" and an individual may be vulnerable of believing inaccurate information. A study involving ten patients with damage to prefrontal cortex, ten patients with damage to other areas of the brain, and sixteen patients who experienced life-threatening medical events but did not suffer any neurological damage, Asp et al. showed that only patients with damage to their prefrontal cortex reported religious fundamentalism. The authors concluded that a normal function of the prefrontal cortex is necessary for psychological doubts and resistance to religious fundamentalism.[21]

The Serotonin Hypothesis of Religion

Lionel Tiger, the Charles Darwin Professor of Anthropology at Rutgers University, and distinguished neuroscientist Michael McGuire in their book *God's Brain* hypothesized that humans are affected by unavoidable sources of stress in daily life, described as "brain pain."[22] To cope with this affliction humans seek secretion of serotonin (a neurotransmitter derived from tryptophan; serotonin deficiency may cause depression) to sooth the brain. Religious beliefs are an evolutionary drive to seek secretion of serotonin which provides the feeling of well-being. Attending a religious service can induce release of a cocktail of neurotransmitters including serotonin. Tiger commented that religion in this sense becomes a self-created, self-consumed endeavor that is soothing for the brain. Therefore, neurological response to religion serves a biological need for humans because in its absence a person may feel depressed. For example, in France where Church attendance is relatively low compared to other European countries, consumption of antidepressant medications is highest among all European countries.[22] The lack of Church attendance could easily factor into the ratio of depression in France.

Serotonin and Enlightenment Experience of Buddha

Serotonin may have played a crucial role in the enlightenment experience of Siddhartha Goutam (Buddha). Siddhartha was born 2500 years ago in Lumbini, Nepal as a son of Shuddhodhana, the king of Kapilavastu and his queen Mayadevi. After his birth astrologers predicted that Siddhartha would reject the comfort of materialistic life of a prince and would seek enlightenment. As a result king Suddhodhana restricted movement of prince Siddhartha outside his palace. When Siddhartha had grown to a wise, intelligent man, he traveled out of his palace to take a tour. He observed a very old man who could barely walk, a sick man in severe pain, and a corpse. He realized pain and death are inevitable in life. When Suddhodhana found out he arranged Siddhartha to marry a beautiful princess, Yosodhara, and later Siddhartha fathered a son named Rahul. However, at the age of twenty-nine, Siddhartha left his wife and son in order to seek an answer to human sufferings.

Renouncing life as a prince to seek enlightenment, Siddhartha searched out and studied under various ascetics, but despite mastering each technique he did not achieve his desired enlightenment. He experimented with various methods of meditation, mind control, breathing techniques (pranayama), and sensory withdrawal, but enlightenment was still unattainable. Finally he practiced extreme fasting until his daily diet was a cup of soup. Siddhartha's body exhibited symptoms of starvation but he did not experience enlightenment. Realizing he was near death but did not achieve his goal, he decided to give up fasting. At that time a passerby woman Sujata offered him a bowl of rice pudding containing milk, rice, and sugar. After eating rice pudding Siddhartha sat again under the Bodhi Tree to meditate and effortlessly achieved his desired enlightenment. Siddhartha reported to his disciples that his enlightenment journey lasted probably nine hours. During this journey Siddhartha had many intense visual experiences where he watched his past lives and past lives of others, cycles of birth and death, passing through heaven and hell and various other supernatural events. These experiences shaped his subsequent teachings as Buddha (the enlightened).

Enlightened with his new knowledge, Buddha was initially hesitant to teach, because it could be difficult to explain his experience in a communicable language but later he decided to talk about his experiences. He left the Bodhi Tree and approximately one hundred miles away, he came across five ascetics to whom he preached his first sermon (henceforth known as *Setting in Motion the Wheel of the Dharma)*, in which he explained the Four Noble Truths, Five perceptions, and the Eightfold Path, which became the pillars of Buddhism. The ascetics then became his first disciples and formed the community of monks known as "*Sangha*." Women were admitted to the *Sangha*, and all barriers of class, race, sex, and previous background were ignored. Only consideration for joining *Sangha* was strong desire to achieve enlightenment and to break the cycle of birth and death. Buddha preached his teachings of overcoming human desires, which are sources of human sufferings, in order to achieve a stage of detachment from material. Buddha preached his teachings for forty-five years to his many disciples and also to both noble and common people. Buddha died at the age of eighty in Kushinagar, India approximately 483 BC.

Paul Joseph published an interesting hypothesis explaining the enlightenment experience of Siddhartha from known neurochemical principles.[23] The hypothesis is that Siddhartha experienced a known medical phenomenon termed as "refeeding syndrome" in which the specific content of the food (rice pudding containing high tryptophan and high carbohydrate, but low protein) he ate played a key role in his enlightenment experience. L-monoamine oxidases (MAO) are a family of enzymes that play key roles in breaking down many neurotransmitters including serotonin. It is well documented in medical literature that starvation is associated with the inhibition of MAO enzymatic activities. For Siddhartha, intense fasting inhibited his MAO activity, but eating rice pudding constituted an intake of dietary tryptophan and carbohydrate from milk and rice. When Siddhartha ate the rice pudding (approximately 250 grams) which contained approximately thirteen grams of tryptophan, sixty-nine grams of carbohydrate, but low in protein, carbohydrates triggered an insulin release, which eventually (through a complex mechanism) increased the tryptophan level in his brain. The tryptophan in the brain of Siddhartha was then converted into serotonin. Because Siddhartha's MAO activity was inhibited due to prolonged starvation, serotonin generated in his brain following eating rice pudding did not degrade due to poor activity of MAO. As a result, excess serotonin in Siddhartha's brain may be responsible for his experience of enlightenment. As a part of initiation, some Hindu monks (sadhus) may have to practice eating small quantities of barley, vegetables, and milk, which are all rich in tryptophan and carbohydrates but low in protein. Therefore, spiritual experiences during such food restriction periods may be due to an accumulation of excess serotonin in the brain.

Religious behavior varies widely among individuals and recent research indicates that such interindividual differences could be explained by neurobiological and genetic factors. Serotonergic neurons are found in all major regions of the human brain and there are fourteen different serotonin receptors that modulate serotonin levels in the brain. The most widely studied receptor is the 5-HT_{1A} receptor which plays an important role in regulating serotonergic activity in the brain. On the basis of PET (positron emission tomography) it has been demonstrated that the 5-HT_{1A} receptor density varies among different people. Borg et al. using fifteen male subjects studied the correlation between the serotonin system and spiritual experiences by mapping the 5-HT_{1A} receptor density in brain using PET technology. The authors observed that the 5-HT_{1A} receptor density was inversely correlated with scores of self-transcendence, a personality trait covering religious behaviors and attitudes. Individuals with high spiritual acceptance scores showed low density of 5-HT_{1A} receptor, which may be associated with higher serotonin release in the brain. The authors concluded that the serotonin system may serve as a biological basis of religious/spiritual experience.[24]

Dopamine, Other Neurotransmitters, and Religion

Review of neurochemistry of dreaming, hallucination, religious beliefs, and religious experiences in normal humans indicates that neurotransmitter dopamine levels are increased in the cortical area of the brain during such experience. Another neurotransmitter, acetylcholine is elevated during dreaming but is decreased during hallucination. The level of norepinephrine is probably decreased during religious behaviors. Therefore, elevated dopamine levels in the cortex and striatum (subcortical part of the forebrain) play a major role in religious experiences.

The four psychiatric disorders most studied in terms of religious activities are bipolar disorder (mania/hypomania), obsessive compulsive disorder, schizophrenia, and temporal lobe epilepsy. Many symptoms in these diseases resemble religious experiences such as hearing voice in schizophrenia and déjà-vu experience in mania. In general patients with schizophrenia show stronger religious beliefs and report more religious experiences than individuals without psychiatric disorders. The relationship between temporal lobe epilepsy and religiosity has also been well documented in the medical literature. Hyper-religiosity is more commonly associated with left sided temporal lobe epilepsy. Therefore, religiosity is possible due to some amount of activation in the left hemisphere of the brain. In addition, all of these disorders predominately involve over-activation of dopamine in the left hemisphere of the brain and excessive dopamine levels in the brain are observed in all such disorders. Classical symptoms of schizophrenia are due to high dopamine levels in the brain. Based on the similarity between higher dopamine levels in these four disorders and religiosity observed in these patients, Previc commented that the evolution of religion is linked to an expansion of the dopaminergic system during human evolution.[25] Sasaki et al. commented that both dopamine and dopamine receptor genes may be involved in religious experiences.[26]

Is There a God Gene?

Dean Hamer's book *The God Gene: How Faith is Hardwired in Our Genes* proposes that the religiosity of an individual is influenced by the genetic makeup. He proposed that the VMAT2 gene is one of many potential genes that impinge spirituality in a person. One particular variation (polymorphism) in the gene is associated with more spirituality. The VMAT2 gene encodes a vesicular monoamine transporter, which is involved in regulating the levels of neurotransmitters including serotonin, dopamine, and norepinephrine. These neurotransmitters play important roles in regulating the brain activities associated with mystic beliefs.[27] Nilsson et al. reported that certain polymorphism in the 5-HTTLPR gene (serotonin-transporter-linked polymorphic region) and the AP-2 beta gene in men were associated with more spirituality but no such effect was observed in women.[28]

Conclusion

Although scientists attempt to demystify religions as well as spiritual experiences using known theories of neuroscience, there are still many unanswered questions. Therefore, whether our brain is hardwired to create God or hardwired to perceive God is still an open question. Although religious/spiritual experiences have similarities with symptoms of certain mental illness, not all religious or spiritual experiences are related to psychiatric disorders. Furthermore religious beliefs and spirituality may be influenced by genetic makeup, but there is no conclusive evidence of a "God Gene" which assuredly creates and makes humans susceptible to the belief of a God. It has been suggested and accepted by many that indeed the concept of God is beyond the realm of science.

Table 3.1 Functions of various parts of the brain

Part of the Brain	Function
Neocortex	Neocortex (neo means new) is the most recent evolutionary developed part of the brain (giving us all higher learning capacities)
Frontal Lobe	Responsible for our personality, judgment, morality, emotions, speech and writing, problem solving, and motor function
Parietal Lobe	Responsible for our visual perception, spatial perception, sense of touch, pain, and temperature; also helps with comprehension (reading and writing)
Occipital Lobe	Responsible for our vision
Temporal Lobe	Responsible for our memory, hearing, understanding, organization, and speech
Limbic area	Responsible for our emotion
Cerebellum	Responsible for our balance and muscle coordination
Brainstem	Responsible for our breathing, regulation of heart rate, respiration, maintaining body temperature, alertness, and other essential body functions

Table 3.2 Functions of major neurotransmitters in the human brain

Neurotransmitter	Function
Acetylcholine	Acetylcholine was the first discovered neurotransmitter (in 1921). It is mainly involved in stimulating muscles.
Serotonin	Serotonin is an inhibitory transmitter that has a profound effect on mood and emotion. Low levels of serotonin are associated with depression and many psychoactive drugs work by elevating levels of serotonin in the brain. Serotonin also controls sleep and appetite.
Dopamine	Dopamine can act as both an excitatory and an inhibitory neurotransmitter. Dopamine plays an important role in aiding the flow of information to the front part of the brain which is linked to thoughts and emotion. Dopamine is also connected to the reward system of the brain. Problems with producing dopamine may cause Parkinson's Disease.
GABA (Gamma-aminobutyric acid)	GABA is an inhibitory neurotransmitter and has a calming effect. Low GABA levels may produce anxiety and drugs such as valium (diazepam) enhance GABA activity. Lack of GABA in certain parts of the brain may be associated with epilepsy. Alteration of GABA neurotransmission has been observed in schizophrenia.

Table 3.2 cont.

Neurotransmitter	Function
Glutamate	Glutamate, an excitatory neurotransmitter, is the most common neurotransmitter in the central nervous system.
Norepinephrine and Epinephrine	Norepinephrines help to produce epinephrine and both are excitatory neurotransmitters. Low levels of norepinephrine may cause low energy, lack of focus and sleep cycle problems. Epinephrine is also involved in regulating heart rate and blood pressure.

Table 3.3 Evolution of the human brain and the origin of religion

- Approximately two million years ago the brain size of ancient humans was 400-600 cubic centimeters. The modern human brain size is 1200-1600 cubic centimeters. At that time they could not have had a perception of religion.
- Around 800,000 years ago, the average brain size exceeded one thousand cubic centimeters. However, between 800,000 and 200,000 years ago only the brain size of early human was increased, not the body size. A final leap of increased brain size took place approximately 180,000 years ago when prehistoric humans had a brain size approaching the brain size of modern humans.
- Approximately 500,000 years ago the human brain was evolved enough in size and complexity that the primitive concept of religion could be conceived.
- There is some evidence that early humans around 150,000 years ago, started pair bonding and practicing monogamy. This could have been related to religious values and moral obligations.
- The limbic system of the human brain was developed enough 30,000-100,000 years ago to experience religious/spiritual experience.

Fig 1. Human Brain: courtesy of Andres Quesada, MD

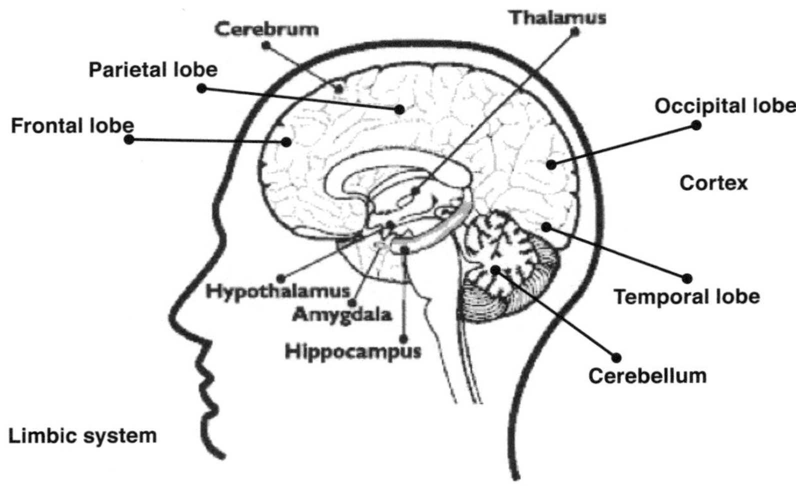

Chapter 4
Scientific Evidence Showing the Health Benefits of Yoga

Introduction

Yoga represents a system of movement and breathing exercises intended to foster a mind-body connection. Yoga is an ancient practice from India. The practice of yoga includes postures (asanas) and breathing exercises (pranayamas), but in addition to yoga, a person is also encouraged to practice meditation, chanting mantras and changing diet (for example eating vegetarian food) with an overall goal of spiritual progress. It is important to note that yoga is a non-denominational practice and anyone can do yoga because faith in Hinduism is not required for such practice. Moreover, yoga can also be practiced only to obtain health benefits, spiritual growth may not be the goal of an individual who is practicing yoga. In this chapter, health benefits of yoga (asana and pranayama) are discussed. In Chapter 5 the physical and mental health benefits of meditation are addressed.

The practice of yoga was introduced by several popular yoga teachers (gurus) to the West between the 1930s and the 1970s but soon after its introduction, yoga became a popular practice in the West. A 1997 study showed that 3.7% Americans practiced yoga, but a 2002 study showed that 5.1% Americans practice yoga. It also showed that Americans who practice yoga are predominately Caucasians (85%) and female (76%) with a mean age of 39.5 years. People who practice yoga, according to the study, are likely to be college educated and most people practice yoga for improving musculoskeletal conditions (body aches and pain) or mental condition. A majority of yoga users (61%) reported that yoga helped them maintain good health and are also non-smokers.[1] According to another survey, an estimated 15.8 million Americans practice yoga and another 9.4 million people reported a strong intention to practice yoga within the next year. Nearly half of the respondents who practiced yoga reported that they initiated practice of yoga with a goal of improving overall health. In some cases a physician or a health care professional recommend them to try yoga. From an economic point of view yoga generates approximately 5.7 billion dollars of annual business in the U.S., ranging from yoga instructions, training, apparel, media, and equipment.[2]

The National Center for Complementary and Integrated Health, a part of National Institute of Health considers yoga as a part of complementary and integrated health approach used by many Americans. Although the most common complementary and integrated health approach among Americans is taking dietary supplements (herbal medicines), yoga is the third most popular complementary and integrated approach among Americans and yoga is more popular than visiting a chiropractor, eating a special diet, getting a massage, or consulting with a homeopathy doctor. Yoga practice is also more popular than meditation. One advantage of yoga is it is safe and effective and has no negative side effects, which is a major concern of some natural remedies.

Yoga and Pranayama

Yoga is a psychosomatic practice with a goal of achieving harmony between the body and mind. "Yoga" is a Sanskrit word meaning *connection* or *union*. The goal of yoga is to integrate the body and the mind through postures (Asana) and breathing methods (Pranayama). Pranayama is derived from two Sanskrit words; "prana" means *life energy* and "ayama" means *prolonging*. Therefore, pranayama means *prolonging life's energy*. The practice of meditation and the practice of yoga both originated at the same time during the Vedic period, in many occasions yoga was combined with meditation to achieve spiritual growth.

There are different types of yoga, but in the U.S., Hatha Yoga is most commonly practiced yoga. It is estimated that approximately

7.4 million Americans practice Hatha Yoga.[3] This type of yoga is relatively easy to learn and it is suitable for a beginner. Hatha Yoga is a gentle practice where an individual moves slowly from one posture to another and during such postures breathing is also regulated. Vinyasa Yoga is a practice similar to Hatha Yoga where postures flow together and are synchronized with breathing. Iyengar Yoga (founded by B.K.S Iyengar) is also widely practiced in U.S. and has some similarity with Hatha Yoga.

Bikram Yoga (founded by Bikram Choudhury) is also popular in U.S., but a major difference between Bikram Yoga and other forms of yoga is that Bikram Yoga is practiced in a hot room where temperature may be as high as 105°F. The idea is that such elevated temperatures may result in more muscle relaxation and sweating may cleanse the body from toxins. Astanga Yoga is a more aggressive form of workout involving various postures where an individual may move quickly from one to another. Ashtanga Yoga (founded by Pattabhi Jois) is also known as Power Yoga, but principles as well as name were derived from the Yoga Sutra of Patanjali. Pattabhi Jois modernized the concept of original Ashtanga (Sanskrit meaning *eight limbs*) Yoga for adaptation in today's practice of yoga.

In Kundalini Yoga, both postures and breathing exercises are practiced at the same time. The goal of Kundalini Yoga is enlightenment. "Kundalini energy" is located at the base of the spine so that female energy, *Shakti,* can move through the spine so that Kundalini can be united with male energy, *Shiva,* located at the head or the Crown Chakra. When such union takes place, a practitioner achieves total enlightenment and nothing in the universe is unknown to the person. However, in reality, this does not happen to most practitioners, but still is a good practice to derive health benefits and spiritual growth. Although original Kundalini Yoga has origins in the ancient texts of Tantra, in 1968, Yogi Bhajan introduced his own version of Kundalini Yoga combining his own teachings with yogic posture, Tantric theories and mantras (chanting). This is also a popular form of yoga practiced in U.S. There are other types of yoga which are also practiced in U.S. These include Sivananda Yoga (founded by Swami Sivananda), Kripula Yoga (founded by Swami Kripalu), Integral Yoga (founded by Swami Satchidananda) and Viniyoga (founded by T.K.V Desikachar). Various types of commonly practiced yoga are listed in Table 4.1.

Pranayama uses breathing exercises to synchronize the flow of energy (prana) through subtle energy channels throughout the body. Although as many as 350,000 energy channels may be present in the human body, the three major energy channels present in the body are *ida* (present in the left nostril), *pingala* (present in the right nostril), and *shusumna* (running through the spinal cord). Proper practice of breathing harmonizes the energy flow of these channels, resulting in excellent health and spiritual growth.[4]

Yoga Versus Exercise

From a broader point of view, yoga is a form of exercise. As we know exercise is very effective in reducing the risk of various cardiovascular diseases including heart attack because regular exercises can increase the level of good cholesterol, decrease blood pressure as well as the level of blood sugar.[5] Interestingly the practice of yoga is similarly effective in reducing risk of hypertension, diabetes, and high cholesterol as other forms of exercise. However, an additional benefit of yoga is improving mood, de-stressing, and lowering the level of anxiety.

Streeter et al. divided health subjects into two groups. The fifteen yoga subjects practiced yoga for sixty minutes, three times a week for twelve weeks while the fifteen control subjects walked for sixty minutes, three times a week for two weeks. Participants in both yoga and walking were metabolically matched to burn similar amounts of calories. The authors observed that the twelve week yoga intervention was associated with greater improvement of mood and reduced anxiety compared to subjects of the walking group. In addition, the authors observed significantly increased gamma-aminobutyric acid (GABA, an important neurotransmitter in the brain) levels in the brain of subjected who practiced yoga and a positive correlation was found between GABA levels in the brain and improved mood as well as a reduced level of anxiety in subjects who practiced yoga.[6] GABA is like the brain's own antidepressant.

Rigorous exercise is practiced by many people including body builders and athletes to improve endurance and muscle strength. However, such rigorous exercises are focused only on the human body and may be competitive in nature. In contrast, yoga is a mind-body integration exercise which is non-competitive in nature. During rigorous exercise the sympathetic nervous system dominates while during yoga the parasympathetic nervous system is activated similar to the practice of meditation. In addition, the risk of injury is significantly lower with the practice of yoga compared to rigorous exercise. Therefore, depending on the goal a person may select rigorous exercise or yoga or even a combination of the two. Rigorous exercise significantly increases the oxidative stress of the body while the practice of yoga increases antioxidant capacity of the body. Major differences between rigorous exercise and yoga are summarized in Table 4.2.

Major Benefits of the Practice of Yoga

Regular practice of yoga is associated with overall good health and mental peace. Stress is related to many diseases but yoga is very effective in reducing stress and restoring antioxidant defense of the body. Yoga improves mood and reduces anxiety level. Yoga is very effective in improving cardiac health because yoga can reduce total cholesterol and at the same time increases HDL-cholesterol (good cholesterol) in blood. The practice of yoga is very beneficial to patients with hypertension (high blood pressure), diabetes, and with previous episodes of cardiovascular diseases. In an individual who suffered from myocardial infarction (heart attack), the practice of yoga may reduce risk of a future heart attack. Yoga is beneficial in patients with eating disorders and may help with weight loss. Yoga is helpful in reducing symptoms of asthma.

Yoga is more effective than exercise in reducing back pain including lower back pain. Yoga may also reduce overall perception of pain and may reduce pain in patients suffering from rheumatoid arthritis and osteoarthritis. Yoga may also reduce the risk of migraine attack. Yoga may shorten labor duration and also may improve birth outcome. Yoga can improve sleep quality and reduce incidence of insomnia. Major health benefits of yoga are listed in Table 4.3.

Yoga Reduces Stress, Depression, and Anxiety

Stress is linked with many diseases (see Chapter 5) and effective stress reduction may significantly reduce risks of many illnesses including cardiovascular diseases and cancer. Similar to meditation, yoga is helpful for stress reduction. Mental health professionals experience high levels of work-related stress which may eventually cause burn-out. Lin et al. divided sixty mental health professionals into two groups. One group participated in a weekly, sixty-minute practice of yoga and the other group relaxed for one hour during tea time (control group). After twelve weeks of intervention, the authors reported significant reduction in work-related stress in the yoga group compared to the control group. The authors concluded that offering a regular yoga class is a viable strategy for work-related stress reductions in healthcare professionals.[7] In another study involving twenty-four women who perceived themselves to be emotionally stressed, Michalsen et al. observed that women who participated in two weekly, ninety-minute Iyengar Yoga classes for three months showed significant improvements on measures or stress and psychological outcome compared to women who did not participate in yoga classes (control group).[8]

Exercise is also effective in reducing the stress and symptoms of depression. Smith et al. divided eighty-one undergraduate students who experienced moderate depression, anxiety, and/or stress into three groups; integrated yoga, exercise, and control. Although participants in both integrated yoga and exercise group experienced decreased depression and reduced stress levels compared to the control group, only participants in the integrated yoga group experienced decreased anxiety and decreased salivary cortisol from the beginning to the end of the study. Cortisol is a hormone which is increased as a response to stress and decreased cortisol level is a biochemical marker of stress reduction. The authors concluded that yoga, which has both ethical and spiritual elements may provide additional benefits over exercise for stress reduction.[9] Batista et al. used twenty-two volunteers to demonstrate that six weeks of Tantric Yoga (fifty minutes per session, twice a week) resulted in significant decreases in salivary cortisol levels indicating that the practice of yoga is effective in reducing stress.[10]

In another study, the authors investigated the effect of Iyengar yoga on twenty-eight volunteers (ages 18–29) who experienced mild depression but were not taking any medication during the study. These subjects did not have any significant yoga experience before the study. The subjects were divided into two groups. One group participated in two one-hour yoga classes each week for five weeks while another group served as the control. The authors reported that subjects of the yoga group demonstrated significant decreases in self-reported symptoms of depression and trait anxiety compared to the control group.[11] Berger et al. studied the effect of yoga on inner-city children's well-being and observed that children participating in yoga (one hour per week for twelve weeks) reported fewer negative reactions in response to stress compared to children who did not participate in yoga. Yoga also improved overall wellbeing in these children.[12] In another study involving sixty-three middle aged women, between the ages of forty and sixty years old, the authors observed that participation in a ninety-minute Hatha Yoga program for eight weeks was associated with significantly reduced perception of stress. The authors concluded that Hatha Yoga is an effective approach for stress reduction.[13]

Yoga Reduces Oxidative Stress and Improves Body's Antioxidant Defense

"Oxygen Paradox" is defined as the fact that any aerobic organisms (organism that cannot survive without oxygen, such as human) require oxygen for survival, but oxygen is also inherently dangerous for these organisms because free radicals such as superoxide radical, hydrogen peroxide, and extremely reactive hydroxyl radicals are commonly produced in our cells during cellular metabolism involving oxygen. In order to survive in an unfriendly oxygen environment living organisms generate water and lipid soluble compounds which can neutralize these dangerous free radicals. These compounds are known as "antioxidants." Several enzymes such as superoxide dismutase, catalase and glutathione peroxidase can deactivate free radicals and are known as antioxidant enzymes. Vitamin C and E are excellent antioxidant. For healthy living a delicate balance must be maintained between oxidative stress and antioxidant defense of the body. Therefore, the reduction of oxidative stress is a goal for healthy living. Boosting antioxidant defense of the body is a good way of reducing oxidative stress.[14]

If the body's antioxidant mechanism does not operate optimally, excess free radicles not neutralized by the body can cause increased oxidative stress. Excess oxidative stress can cause damage to many bio-molecules of our body including lipids, proteins, carbohydrates, and even DNA. Many diseases are linked to oxidative stress including cardiovascular diseases, diabetes, neurodegenerative diseases (Parkinson and Alzheimer's disease), inflammatory bowel disease, ulcerative colitis, cancer, and others. Living a stressful life increases oxidative stress. However, regular yoga practice can reduce oxidative stress by increasing the antioxidant defense of the body. Another approach of increasing the antioxidant defense of the body is to include fruits and vegetables in every day diet. Fruits and vegetables contain numerous phytochemicals that are excellent antioxidants. In addition, fruits and vegetables contain antioxidant vitamins.[14]

Several published papers in medical literature indicate that practice of yoga improves antioxidant defense of the body. Yadav et al. conducted a study using 104 subjects (fifty-nine males and forty-five females) who participated in a yoga based lifestyle modification program (nine days outpatient program consisting of a one-hour practice of yoga and educational videos on yoga) demonstrated that serum concentrations of malondialdehyde (end product of lipid peroxidation which is considered an excellent biological marker of oxidative stress) as measured by thiobarbituric acid reactive substances (TBARS) decreased significantly after nine days of yoga practice. The mean initial concentration of TBRAS in these subjects was 1.72 nmol/ml but after participation in yoga program the mean TBRAS value decreased to 1.57 nmol/ml. The authors concluded that yoga reduces oxidative stress by boosting antioxidant defense of the body.[15]

Sinha et al. divided fifty-one healthy male volunteers into two groups; one group of thirty participated in a six month yoga program while the twenty-one volunteers of the control group were engaged in exercise for the same six month period. After six months, the authors observed significantly increased total antioxidant capacity of blood in volunteers who participated in the yoga program compared to the control group. Blood level of reduced glutathione, an antioxidant was also increased significantly in volunteers who participated in the yoga program compared to volunteers in the control group indicating that yoga improves the antioxidant status of the body.[16] In another study based on sixty-four physically trained male volunteers, Pal et al. observed that practice of yoga for three months significantly increased levels of vitamin C, vitamin E and reduced glutathione (all are antioxidants) in blood of volunteers who participated in the yoga program compared to volunteers of the control group who participated in physical training. In addition, total antioxidant capacity of the blood was also significantly increased in volunteers who participated in the yoga training compared to volunteers who were engaged in physical training. The authors concluded that yoga improves antioxidant defense of the body and is superior to exercise.[17]

Yoga Reduces Perception of Pain in Various Musculoskeletal Diseases

Pain is the major symptom of various musculoskeletal diseases. Musculoskeletal pain, which is more common among elderly people, may be caused by damage to muscles, bones, joints, ligaments, and even nerve. Arthritis is another common musculoskeletal disorder. Some musculoskeletal disorders, such as carpal tunnel syndrome, cause pain by compressing nerves. Yoga is helpful in reducing symptoms of various musculoskeletal diseases.

Chronic lower back pain is the most common form of pain and an estimated twenty-seven to thirty million people in the U.S. may suffer from such pain. Tekur et al. studied the effect of yoga intervention on people experiencing chronic lower back pain using eighty subjects (thirty-seven females and forty-three males). The people assigned to the yoga group received instructions for performing certain postures (asanas) and pranayama and practiced yoga for seven days. The subjects in the control group received physical therapy. The authors observed that seven days of the intensive residential yoga program reduced pain, anxiety, and depression as well as improved spinal mobility of people with lower back pain more effectively than subjects who participated in physiotherapy exercises [18]. In a systematic review of ten studies involving a total 967 chronic back pain patients, Cramer et al. concluded that there is a strong evidence for short term effectiveness and moderate evidence for long term effectiveness of yoga in treating chronic lower back pain. Therefore, yoga can be recommended as an additional therapy to treat patients with chronic lower back pain [19]. In addition to alleviating lower back pain, yoga is effective in reducing the general perception of pain. Based on review of ten clinical trials, Posadzki et al. concluded that yoga has a potential for effective pain management.[20]

Yoga is effective in reducing pain in patients suffering from arthritis. Approximately 21% of adults suffer from arthritis. Moonaz et al. studied the effect of yoga intervention on patients with arthritis using seventy-five sedentary adults who either suffer from rheumatoid arthritis or knee osteoarthritis. Both types of arthritis cause joint pain, but ostearthritis is more common than rheumatoid arthritis. The main difference between osteoarthritis and rheumatoid arthritis is the cause behind the joint pain. In rheumatoid arthritis, the body's own immune system degenerates the joints (autoimmune disease) while osteoarthritis is caused by mechanical wear and tear on joints. Moonaz and his colleagues randomly assigned subjects either to a yoga intervention group (two sixty-minute classes and one home practice per week for eight weeks) or to a waitlist. After eight weeks, subjects in the yoga group had better waking capacity, positive attitude, and lower scores on the depression scale compared to subjects in the waiting list. Subjects in the yoga group even showed overall improvement in quality of life. The authors concluded that yoga may help sedentary individuals with arthritis to safely increase physical activity, and improve physical and psychological wellbeing.[21] Sharma, based on review of nine studies dealing with effectiveness of yoga on alleviating pain in arthritis, concluded that yoga appears to be a promising complementary and alternative medicine modality for treating arthritis.[22]

Fibromyalgia is a chronic syndrome characterized by widespread pain, sleep disturbance, stiffness, fatigue, headache and mood disorder. Hennard had eleven participants with fibromyalgia participate in an eight week yoga and meditation intervention, which significantly improved overall health status of these individuals due to decreased stiffness, anxiety, and depression. Significant improvements were also observed in number of days "felt good" and number of days "missed work: due to fibromyalgia."[23] In another study involving ten patients suffering from fibromyalgia (ages 39–64), Rudrud observed that participation in an eight week Hatha Yoga program (instructions were provided twice a week) was associated with significant reductions in symptoms of fibromyalgia.[24]

Carpal-tunnel syndrome is a compressive neuropathy (nerve pain) of the median nerve which runs from the forearm into the palm of the hand. The carpal tunnel is a narrow, rigid passageway of ligament and bones at the base of the hand through which median nerve passes. Sometimes, thickening from irritated tendons or other swelling narrows the tunnel and causes the median nerve to be compressed which results in nerve pain causing a burning sensation. This disorder is more common in women than men. This syndrome is commonly associated with rheumatoid arthritis, diabetes, hypothyroidism and other conditions.[25]

Yoga based intervention is helpful in reducing symptoms of carpal-tunnel syndrome. In one study involving forty-two individuals (ages 24–77) with carpal-tunnel syndrome, the authors divided subjects into two groups. Subjects in one group participated in yoga based intervention (consisting of eleven postures designed for strengthening, stretching and balancing each joints in the upper body) which lasted for eight weeks (twice weekly) and subjects of another group wore wrist splints to supplement their current treatment. The authors observed that subjects in the yoga group had significant improvement in grip strength and also experienced reduced pain compared to the control group. Moreover, subjects in the yoga group also showed improvement in Phalen sign (Phalen sign or Phalen maneuver is a test used in diagnosis of carpal-tunnel syndrome. This test involves several wrist maneuvers and improvement in Phalen sign indicates that the disease is responding to therapy). The authors concluded that yoga intervention is more effective than conventional wrist splinting in relieving symptoms of carpal-tunnel syndrome.[26]

Yoga Reduces Risk of Cardiovascular Diseases, Including Heart Attack

Cardiovascular diseases including heart attacks (myocardial infarction) are the leading cause of morbidity and mortality throughout the world. Cardiovascular diseases may be related to electrical malfunction of the heart or coronary artery disease which is related to narrowing of coronary arteries due to deposit of cholesterol particles within walls of the artery that eventually develop into plaques (this process is called atherosclerosis) that restrict blood flow to the heart. When blood flow to the heart is severally inhibited or stopped due to plaque and blood clots, a heart attack may result. Coronary artery disease (also called ischemic heart disease, atherosclerotic heart disease or coronary heart disease) is a group of diseases including stable angina, unstable angina (chest pain), heart attack, and sudden coronary death.

Numerous studies have demonstrated a link between elevated cholesterol levels and risk of cardiovascular diseases. In the large international INTERHEART study, abnormal lipid profile and smoking were shown to be the two most important risk factors for cardiovascular diseases. Other important risk factors are hypertension, obesity, and diabetes.[27] Risk factors for cardiovascular diseases can be either un-modifiable risk factors or modifiable ones. These risk factors are summarized in Table 4.4. According to World Health Organization (WHO), the majority of cardiovascular diseases can be prevented by risk factor modification and changing lifestyle. Unfortunately approximately 70% of Americans are overweight and fewer than 15% of children and adults exercise sufficiently. 11–13% of American adults have diabetes and 34% have hypertension, indicating the depth of the problem and risk of cardiovascular diseases in Americans.[28]

Relation between serum or plasma (after centrifugation of blood, the upper layer which is mostly water and slightly yellow in color is called serum or plasma depending on if no anticoagulant or anticoagulant is present in the blood collection tube) cholesterol and risk for arthrosclerosis (narrowing of coronary arteries due to plaque buildup) has been extensively investigated by the Framingham Heart Study. This study was initiated in 1948 in Framingham, Massachusetts by enrolling 5,209 men and women to study risk factors for heart diseases. The study was under the direction of National Heart Institute now known as National Heart, Lung, and Blood Institute. Many important guidelines regarding the risk of cardiovascular diseases emerged from Framingham Heart Study.

Initial results of the Framingham study established the link between high total cholesterol and low HDL-cholesterol (high density lipoprotein cholesterol, also known as good cholesterol) as two major risk factors for cardiovascular diseases. However, later reports observed the link between elevated triglycerides and higher risk of cardiovascular diseases. Currently the basis of treatment of lipid disorders is the third report of the expert panel of the National Cholesterol Education program and currently desirable total cholesterol level of less than 200 mg/dL (dL stands for 100 milliliter) has been universally accepted. Any serum cholesterol above 240 mg/dL is associated with high risk of cardiovascular diseases. Similarly HDL-cholesterol below 40 mg/dL is associated with higher risk of cardiovascular diseases. Serum triglyceride should be below 150 mg/dL. Highly elevated triglyceride over 500 mg/dL is associated with higher risk of cardiovascular diseases. Unfortunately, in U.S. approximately 16.3% of the population suffer from high cholesterol levels of 240 mg/dL or higher. This population has a cardiovascular risk factor twice as high as people with optimal cholesterol level of 200 mg/dL or lower. In 2007 nearly one-fifth of Americans reported that their cholesterol level had not been checked in last five years [29]. Yoga reduces risk of cardiovascular diseases (including heart attack) by lowering serum cholesterol level and improving level of HDL-cholesterol. Increased oxidative stress is also associated with higher risk of cardiovascular diseases. Yoga significantly reduces oxidative stress thus lowering risk of cardiovascular diseases including heart attack[30].

Studies indicate that yoga may reduce total cholesterol, low-density lipoprotein cholesterol (LDL cholesterol or bad cholesterol), and triglycerides level in serum or plasma. Whether yoga may increase HDL-cholesterol (good cholesterol) is controversial with some studies reporting increased level of HDL-cholesterol due to practice of yoga while other studies found no change in HDL-cholesterol level. However, a recent study by Yadav et al. indicates that even short term yoga is helpful in improving serum HDL-cholesterol level. The study included 238 volunteers (Average age of thirty-nine) who participated in a ten day yoga based lifestyle intervention program. HDL-cholesterol levels increased more significantly in volunteers who had initially low HDL-cholesterol.[31] Mayor commented that yoga can significantly reduce cardiovascular risk factors by reducing body mass index, blood pressure, and LDL-cholesterol (bad cholesterol). In addition, yoga can increase HDL-cholesterol level. The author reviewed thirty-seven clinical trials enrolling 2,768 subjects and observed that mean systolic blood pressure was reduced by 5.21 mm Hg (millimeter of mercury), LDL-cholesterol by 12.14 mg/dL while HDL-cholesterol was increased by 3.2 mg/dL.[32] Chu et al. based on meta-analysis of thirty-two studies also observed that yoga can reduce body weight, LDL-cholesterol, total cholesterol, triglycerides, and systolic blood pressure thus significantly reducing risk factors of cardiovascular diseases including heart attack.[33]

Yoga is Helpful in Patients with Type 2 Diabetes

There are two types of diabetes; diabetes mellitus and diabetes insipidus. Diabetes mellitus is a common condition related to either insulin resistance (due to obesity or other factors) or reduced production of insulin. Diabetes insipidus is a an uncommon condition that occurs when kidneys are unable to concentrate urine due to either a lack of secretion of the antidiuretic hormone (cranial diabetes insipidus) or due to the inability of the antidiuretic hormone to work at the collection duct of the kidney (nephrogenic diabetes insipidus). Diabetes mellitus can be due to a lack of insulin secretion and as a result this type of diabetes is known as insulin-dependent diabetes. This type is also called Type 1 Diabetes (juvenile diabetes) because it is diagnosed at young age and treatment is insulin injection. More common is insulin resistant diabetes or Type 2 Diabetes (non-insulin dependent diabetes) which is usually detected at a later age (forty years and older) and represents 90-95% of all diabetes. This type of Diabetes may be treated with oral hypoglycemic agents but for some patients insulin may be needed 5-15 years after diagnosis.

Yoga is helpful for individuals with Type 2 Diabetes because yoga, by lowering body weight, decreases insulin resistance. Type 2 Diabetes is also a risk factor for cardiovascular diseases. Yoga reduces blood pressure and improves serum lipid profile, thus decreases the risk of cardiovascular diseases in patients with diabetes. Whether yoga is effective in reducing blood sugar is controversial. In one study, the authors reported that participating in Hatha Yoga classes three times a week for six weeks had no effect on fasting blood sugar [34]. However, in another study, the authors recruited thirty diabetic (age range: 30-55 years) and thirty non-diabetic patients who participated in daily yoga training every day for six months. Before initiation of yoga practice, the mean fasting glucose in Type 2 Diabetic patients was 154.1 mg/dL. After three months the mean fasting glucose value was reduced to 149.6 mg/dL and after six months the mean fasting glucose value was further reduced to 141.42 mg/dL. In non-diabetic patients the mean fasting glucose value was 84.38 mg/dL. After the initiation of yoga, the mean fasting glucose was 82.14 mg/dL after six months. The authors concluded that yoga is effective in reducing blood sugar in patients with Type 2 Diabetes.[35]

Yoga is Associated with Positive Outcome in Pregnancy

During pregnancy women undergo distinct physiological changes which may often induce psychological stress. The well-being of mothers is critical for a healthy outcome in pregnancy. Maternal stress and anxiety during pregnancy may negatively affect the outcome of pregnancy by affecting the intrauterine environment by altering blood flow and oxygen to the fetus and also by releasing stress hormones from the placenta. Although physical exercise can reduce maternal stress, a mind-body approach such as yoga is more beneficial for pregnant mothers. Moreover, depression and/or anxiety during pregnancy may also negatively affect the outcome of pregnancy. Davis et al., based on a study of forty-six pregnant women with symptoms of depression and anxiety, reported that an eight week yoga intervention was more effective in reducing symptoms of anxiety and depression than traditional therapy.[36]

In general, stress levels in pregnant women increase with gestation age. However, yoga is especially effective in reducing maternal stress during weeks 28–36 of pregnancy. Yoga can also reduce symptoms of pregnancy related discomforts including morning sickness. Moreover, yoga can also reduce perceived pain during labor as well as the duration of labor. Practice of yoga may also increase the birth weight of infants. However, yoga is especially effective in reducing maternal stress from the 28th to 36th week of pregnancy. Yoga also reduces the risk of preterm labor.[37] In a study based on seventy-four pregnant women, divided into two groups, either the experimental group (practiced yoga) or the control group (did not participate in yoga), the authors observed that women who practiced yoga had higher levels of maternal comfort during labor and the two hours post labor. The women who practiced yoga also showed a shorter duration of the first stage of labor as well as an overall shorter total time of labor compared to women in the control group.[38]

Rakshani et al., based on a study of fifty-nine high risk pregnant women who were randomly assigned into a yoga group (one hour per day, three times a week from the 12th to 28th week of gestation) or a control group, observed that fetus in the yoga group at 28th week of gestation had significantly higher head circumference, biparietal diameter (the diameter across the developing fetus's skull), and estimated fetal weight compared to women in the control group. The authors concluded that yoga can improve the intrauterine fetal growth and the utero-fetal placental circulation in women with high risk pregnancy.[39]

Yoga Improving Quality of Life in Cancer Patients

The practice of yoga improves quality of life in cancer patients by reducing stress, improving coping skills and by increasing spiritual awareness. Yoga may also help patients suffering from breast cancer. In one study which included fourteen breast cancer patients, Sudarshan et al. observed that participation in a weekly, one hour yoga program for twelve weeks, significantly reduced anxiety, depression and pain symptoms in these women. In addition, both right and left shoulder abduction and flexibility also improved in these individuals.[40] Up to 50% of breast cancer survivors receiving hormone therapy (aromatase inhibitors or tamoxifen) report muscle and joint pain. Peppone et al., based on a study of seventy-two breast cancer survivors receiving tamoxifen and ninety-five survivors receiving aromatase inhibitors, showed that four weeks of yoga intervention (seventy-five-minute session, twice per week) significantly reduced muscle ache, perception of pain and overall total physical discomfort.[41] Yoga is an effective, well-tolerated exercise intervention in reducing insomnia and improving sleep quality in patients with various types of cancer.[42]

Yoga Reduces Symptoms in Asthma Patients and Patients with COPD

Asthma is a chronic inflammatory disorder of reversible airway obstruction affecting approximately twenty-four million Americans and three hundred million people worldwide. The chronic inflammation causes blocking of airways producing symptoms such as wheezing, breathlessness, chest tightness, and coughing at night or early morning. Yoga is effective in improving pulmonary functions and quality of life in asthma patients. Sodhi et al. using 120 non-smoking male and female asthma patients (ages 17-50) showed that the practice of yoga breathing exercise for eight weeks was associated with a reduced number of asthma attacks per week as well as a reduction of dosage of medication needed by such asthma patients. The authors concluded that yoga breathing exercise used adjunctively with standard medical care significantly improved the quality of life in asthma patients.[43]

Agnihorty et al. based on a study using 241 subjects (120 subjects participated in yoga plus standard medical care and 121 control subjects receiving only standard medical care) showed that six months of yoga intervention (thirty minutes per day) was associated with significant improvement of quality of life as well as biochemical parameters in asthma patients. Hemoglobin increased by a mean of 7.52% in patients who participated in yoga. Eosinophils play crucial role in asthma attack because activation of the eosinophils is associated with asthma attack. In general, patients who have fatal asthma attacks show significantly elevated level of blood eosinophils than people who suffer from chronic asthma. Yoga is very effective in reducing eosinophils as authors reported a 48% decrease of blood eosinophils level in asthma patients who participated in six months of yoga intervention. Monocytes also accumulate in airways during asthma attack. Yoga also reduced monocytes by 63% in blood. The antioxidant status of asthma patients was also improved after yoga intervention as evidenced by a 5% increase in the serum superoxide dismutase enzyme level (antioxidant enzyme). Free radicals increase symptoms of asthma while improved antioxidant defense of the body can alleviate asthma symptoms. The authors concluded that yoga is effective in improving the quality of life as well as biochemical parameters in asthma patients.[44]

Chronic obstructive pulmonary disease (COPD) is an obstructive lung disease characterized by chronically poor airflow to the lungs. The main symptoms are shortness of breath, coughing, and sputum production. Cigarette smoking is a major cause of developing COPD and patients with chronic bronchitis may also develop COPD. Worldwide, COPD affects approximately 330 million people with nearly three million deaths annually. Prevalence of COPD is higher in courtiers with higher prevalence of smoking among people. Yoga is effective in improving quality of life of COPD patients. In one study of twenty-two patients with COPD, six week yoga (one hour session, three times per week) intervention was associated with significant improvements in lung function as well as the quality of life in these patients.[45] Liu et al., based on systematic review and meta-analysis of five randomized clinical trials involving 233 patients suffering from COPD, concluded that yoga significantly improved lung function and exercise capacity in these patients. Therefore, yoga may be considered an adjunct pulmonary rehabilitation program in COPD patients.[46]

Yoga Reduces Symptoms in Patients with Multiple Sclerosis

Multiple sclerosis is a chronic autoimmune disease where the body's immune system (T-cell mediated) mounts an attack on the body's central nervous system (involving brain and the spinal cord) causing devastating effect. Demyelination (damage or destruction of myelin sheet that protects nerve fibers) is responsible for impaired neural conductions as well as many symptoms associated with multiple sclerosis. The onset of disease occurs in young adults (ages 20–40) and the disease is more common in females than in males. Major symptoms include overall feeling of weakness, pain, depression, cognitive impairment, imbalance, fatigue, and depression. There is no known cure of multiple sclerosis and as a result medications are used to slow down the progression of the disease and to maintain the quality of life.

Yoga's focus on movement, breathing, and stretching is helpful in managing symptoms of patients suffering from multiple sclerosis. Approximately 50% of patients with multiple sclerosis suffer from depression and studies have shown that even an eight week yoga intervention is effective in significantly reducing depression among patients with multiple sclerosis. Yoga is also helpful in managing symptoms such as pain, fatigue, spasticity, balance, bladder control, and sexual function in patients suffering from multiple sclerosis[47].

Balance problems and fatigue are two major symptoms of patients with multiple sclerosis. Guner and Inanici discovered through a study of eight multiple sclerosis patients who participated in a twelve week, bi-weekly yoga program that even short term yoga intervention significantly improved balance, step length, and walking speed as well as reduce fatigue among these patients.[48] In another study based on ninety patients who were randomly assigned to a yoga group, aerobics exercise group, or control group, Hassanpour Dehkordi observed that patients assigned in both the yoga and the aerobics exercise groups experienced less fatigue and pain compared to patients in the control group. In addition, patients in both the yoga and the aerobic exercise groups had better physical and emotional status than patients in the control group. The author concluded that both yoga and aerobics exercise could decrease some symptoms of multiple sclerosis as well as therapeutic costs, hospital stays, and days lost from work as well as increasing patient's overall efficiency.[49]

Yoga Improves Sleep Quality and Reduces Insomnia

Yoga is effective in improving sleep quality and may be used as a treatment for chronic insomnia. Khalsa studied the effect of a simple daily yoga treatment as a potential therapy for treating people suffering from chronic insomnia. Participants maintained sleep-wake diaries during two weeks of pretreatment and a subsequent eight weeks of yoga therapy where they practiced yoga on their own. For all twenty participants who completed the study (out of the initial enrollment of 40 participants), yoga practice was associated with significant improvements in sleep efficiency, total sleep time and sleep onset latency.[50]

In general, sleep quality decreases with advanced age and many elderly people suffer from poor sleep quality and often undiagnosed insomnia. If the quality of sleep is poor or if insomnia is untreated it may affect the overall quality of life and may impair daily functions of elderly people. Insomnia is a risk factor for accidents and falls. Based on a study of older men and women (ages greater than sixty), Halpern et al. observed that bi-weekly yoga classes for twelve weeks significantly improved overall quality of sleep, sleep efficiency, sleep latency, and sleep duration in individuals who practiced yoga compared to control subjects. Yoga also improved overall quality of life in these elderly subjects because they experienced lesser depression, anxiety, fatigue, stress, tension, and anger compared to subjects in the control group. Therefore, yoga not only improved sleep quality and physical wellbeing in these subjects but also improved their emotional wellbeing.[51]

Chen et al. divided sixty-nine elderly residents of an assisted living facility into two groups; one group participated in a seventy-minute yoga program three times a week for twenty-four weeks and another group was the control group. After the study period, elderly subjects who participated in the yoga program showed significant improvement in overall sleep quality compared to subjects of the control group. In addition, depression, sleep disturbances, and daytime dysfunctions were significantly decreased in elderly subjects who practiced yoga compared to subjects who did not practice yoga. The authors concluded that a yoga program should be incorporated as an activity in assisted living facilities and other long term care facilities in order to improve sleep quality and decrease depression in elderly residents.[52]

The practice of yoga is also effective in reducing incidence of insomnia in postmenopausal women. In one study involving forty-four postmenopausal women (ages 50–65) who had a diagnosis of insomnia but not undergoing hormonal therapy, the authors observed that four months of yoga intervention resulted in significant reduction in insomnia severity in women belonging to the yoga group compared to women in the passive stretching group (control group). The women who participated in yoga also showed lower menopausal symptoms (hot flashes, dry vagina, mood swing, etc.) and had overall improvement in quality of life. The authors concluded that yoga is effective in reducing menopausal symptoms and insomnia as well as improving overall quality of life in postmenopausal women.[53]

Yoga Reduces Symptoms of Menopause

Managing symptoms of menopause primarily hot flashes by hormone replacement therapy has many side effects. As a result, there is a considerable research to find an alternative to hormone replacement therapy. Several herbal supplements including black cohosh have been implicated for treating symptoms of menopause but even herbal supplements are not free from side effects. Several studies indicate that yoga may be a safe, complementary and alternative modality to reduce symptoms of menopause including hot flashes.

Avis et al. randomized perimenopausal women (2-12 months of amenorrhea) and postmenopausal women (more than twelve months of amenorrhea) aged 45-58 (total number of women studied: fifty-four) who experienced at least four hot flashes a day into one of the three groups: yoga (weekly ninety-minute class), health and wellness education and wait list. The trial lasted for ten weeks and all women kept a personal diary recording incidence of hot flashes. On week ten, women in the yoga group reported a 66% decrease in hot flashes frequency, while women in the control group (waitlisted) reported a 36% decrease in hot flashes frequency. Interestingly, women in the health and wellness education group also experienced a 63% decline in frequency of hot flashes in week ten. The authors concluded that yoga is an effective behavioral option for reducing incidence of hot flashes but may not offer any added advantage over other interventions such as health and wellness education.[54]

Cohen wrote an editorial in the *Menopause* journal citing several studies on effectiveness of yoga in alleviating symptoms of menopause. One of the cited studies was based on 120 postmenopausal women who participated in a weekly sixty-minute yoga session for eight weeks, the authors observed that yoga is effective in reducing symptoms related to menopause. Women in the yoga group also reported experiencing less stress and neuroticism compared to women in the control group. In another study, where women participated in a weekly ninety-minute yoga intervention for eight weeks, it was reported that women in the yoga group experienced approximately 30% reductions in hot flashes frequency compared to the control group. Intensity of hot flashes was also reduced in women of the yoga group. Based on these two studies cited here and other studies, the author summarized that yoga has a beneficial effect on reducing symptoms of menopause. However, more work is also needed in this field.[55]

Yoga may Reduce Tobacco, Alcohol, and Drug Abuse and Help with Drug/Alcohol Rehabilitation

There is evidence supporting the role of yoga in reducing the craving for tobacco, drugs, and alcohol. As a result, yoga can be used as a safe, complementary therapy to a drug and alcohol rehabilitation program in addition to standard care. Elibero et al., based on a study of seventy-six smokers who participated in a thirty-minute exercise protocol (brisk walk on a treadmill) or Hatha Yoga or a non-activity control condition following one hour of nicotine abstinence, observed that subjects who participated in physical activity or Hatha Yoga experienced significant decrease in craving.[56]

Hallgren et al. based on a study of eighteen alcohol-dependent outpatients who either participated in a ten week yoga intervention group (plus usual treatment) or no yoga, reported that alcohol consumption was reduced significantly in participants of the yoga group. The author concluded that larger studies are needed to assess the efficacy of long term effectiveness of yoga as an adjunct treatment for alcohol dependence.[57]

Can Yoga Hurt?

Although injuries from yoga are not commonly reported, injuries do occur. As a result it is preferable to practice yoga with a group or few individuals rather than practicing alone. Based on a report of 2,230 individuals who practice yoga, less than 1% reported injury from yoga that led to discontinuation of it.[58] Russell et al. reported a detailed study involving yoga related injuries in Canada from 1991 to 2010 based on Canadian emergency department reports. A total of sixty-six individuals sustained sixty-seven yoga-related injuries and such injuries were more common among women than men. Sprains were the most commonly reported injury (34%) affecting mostly lower extremities. Russell et al. commented that yoga related injuries requiring emergency care are uncommon.[59] Bikram Yoga is strenuous and practiced in a heated room. Ferrera et al. reported a case of a fifty-three-year-old man without any heart disease who suffered from an acute heart attack (myocardial infarction) during a Bikram Yoga session. He was hospitalized and responded to the treatment, eventually discharged with a full recovery.[60]

Conclusion

Yoga has a history of less than one hundred years in the West. Nevertheless, it has been widely accepted by the general population as an effective, complementary, and integrative health approach for improving general wellbeing as well as an effective modality for reducing stress, depression, and anxiety. Yoga is effective in reducing lower back pain, pain associated with several diseases, symptoms of menopause, and insomnia. Woodway concluded that yoga can be considered as a therapy that is useful in alleviating both physical and emotional pain.[61] Moreover, yogic practices enhance cardiovascular function, promote recovery from and treatment of addiction, reduce stress, anxiety, depression, and chronic pain, improve sleep pattern, and enhance overall well-being and quality of life.

Although yoga can be learned by watching videos, the International Association of Yoga Therapists was founded in 1989 to define yoga therapy and to organizing yoga teachers attempting to use yoga in treating health conditions. This association has published curriculum for yoga teachers suggesting eight hundred hours of study. However, at this point, no formal certification or credential is needed to be a member of the association. Verrastro commented that yoga is a therapy and currently there are good evidences supporting specific use of yoga for lower back pain, depression and anxiety. In addition, there is evidence to support the use of yoga in helping patients with asthma, reducing symptoms of menopause, lowering blood pressure, and improving balance and stability. However, patients with osteoporosis or other risk of fractures should exercise caution for using certain types of yoga protocol [62]. It is wise to initiate the practice of yoga with a yoga teacher or by taking yoga lessons in a group rather than self-learning from books or videos because practicing yoga in the wrong way, like many exercises, may hurt. A seasoned yoga instructor can decide which type of yoga and frequency of yoga practice will be most beneficial for a beginner.

Table 4.1 Various types of yoga

Type of Yoga	Level of Practice	Comments
Hatha Yoga	Gentle practice of yoga suitable for beginners	In Hatha Yoga the focus is on various postures but not on breathing.
Vinyasa Yoga	Gentle to moderate	In this practice an instructor takes a student step by step from beginner's level to higher level of practice. Vinayasa Yoga has some similarity with Hatha Yoga, but is a fluid transition from pose to pose, moving with your breath.
Iyengar Yoga	Gentle practice of yoga suitable for beginners	This consists of various poses which may be held for minutes at a time. Sometimes a yoga belt or yoga pillow may be used to hold the postures.
Bikram Yoga	Very challenging form of yoga	This is a demanding sequence of twenty-six postures and two breathing exercises which are usually practiced in a hot room (temperature may be as high as 105°F and sometimes creeps up higher).
Ashtanga Yoga	Very challenging form of yoga	This is an athletic form of yoga consisting of various postures along with various breathing exercises. The principles as well as name were derived from the Yoga Sutra of Patanjali. Pattabhi Jois modernized the concept of original Ashtanga Yoga for adaptation in today's practice.

Table 4.1 cont.

Type of Yoga	Level of Practice	Comments
Kundalini Yoga	Challenging form of yoga intended for spiritual growth	In Kundalini Yoga the focus is on both postures and controlled breathing (pranayama). Mantras may be repeated during such practice. Although based on the original Tantric practice, Yogi Bhajan has introduced a modern form of Kundalini Yoga.
Sivananda Yoga	Gentle practice of yoga suitable for beginners	This is a gentle sequence of various postures where pranayama and meditation may also be included in the practice.
Kripula Yoga	Gentle practice of yoga suitable for beginners	Postures and breathing awareness are often integrated into this practice. The goal is to achieve mind-body awareness.
Integral Yoga	Gentle practice of yoga suitable for beginners	This type of yoga incorporates various postures with breathing exercises, chanting, and meditation.
Viniyoga	Gentle practice of yoga suitable for beginners	This is a therapeutic and gentle practice of yoga where a teacher may teach an individual student specific postures which will be most suitable for his/her practice.

Table 4.2 Major differences between rigorous exercise and yoga

Rigorous Exercise	Yoga
Significantly increases oxidative stress	Reduces oxidative stress
Competitive and goal oriented	Non-competitive
Develops and tones particular muscle (for example, weight lifting training tones bicep, tricep, and quadricep muscles and increases muscle strength)	Normalizes all muscle tones evenly instead of improving strength or tone of specific muscles
High risk of injuring muscles and/or ligaments	Low risk of muscle or ligament injury
High calorie intake	Low calorie intake
Reduces cholesterol, blood sugar, and blood pressure, but has no effect on reducing anxiety	Reduces cholesterol, blood sugar, and blood pressure, and has many mental health benefits including reducing stress and anxiety
Sympathetic nervous system is stimulated	Parasympathetic nervous system is stimulated
It may be difficult for elderly to participate in rigorous exercise	Age is not a bar for practicing yoga because there are gentler methods for different needs and abilities
No spiritual growth	Regular practice of yoga and meditation results in spiritual growth

Table 4.3 Major health benefits of yoga

- Reduced stress (reduced level of cortisol, a stress hormone), anxiety, and depression
- Reduced oxidative stress and improved the antioxidant defense of the body
- Reduced perception of pain in various musculoskeletal diseases (lower back pain, rheumatoid arthritis, osteoarthritis, fibromyalgia, and carpal tunnel syndrome)
- Reduced risk of cardiovascular diseases including heart attack
- Helpful in patients with type 2 diabetes
- Associated with positive outcome in pregnancy
- Improved quality of life in some cancer patients
- Reduced symptoms in asthma patients and patients with COPD
- Reduced symptoms in patients with multiple sclerosis
- Improved sleep quality and reduced incidences of insomnia
- Reduced symptoms of menopause
- May reduce tobacco, alcohol and drug abuse and help with drug/alcohol rehabilitation

Table 4.4 Various risk factors for cardiovascular diseases including heart attacks

Un-modifiable Risk Factors	Modifiable Risk Factors
• Male sex • Advanced age (male >45 years; female >55 years) • Postmenopausal • Family history (myocardial infarction of sudden death below fifty-five years of age in father or other male first degree relative or below sixty-five years of age in mother or other first degree female relative) • Genetic factors (African Americans, Mexican Americans, Native Indians, people from Indian subcontinent have higher risk of heart diseases than Caucasians) • Genetically inherited high blood cholesterol due to LDL-receptor defect* (familial hypercholesterolemia)	• Abnormal lipid profile due to lifestyle • Hypertension (controlling hypertension reduces the risk) • Diabetes (controlling blood sugar reduces the risk) • Smoking • Obesity • Physical inactivity • Excessive use of alcohol (moderate drinking** protects against cardiovascular diseases and stroke, but excessive drinking increases risks of such diseases) • Poor diet (no fruits and vegetables but high carbohydrate intake) • Excessive stress • Uncontrolled anger

*LDL (low density cholesterol) receptors present in the liver remove low density lipoprotein cholesterol which is also known as bad cholesterol from blood.

**Moderate drinking is up to two alcoholic drinks per day for men and up to one alcoholic drink per day for women

Chapter 5

The Physical and Mental Health Benefits of Meditation

Introduction

Meditation is an ancient tradition of training the human mind in order to achieve a very relaxed state of being where thoughts are filtered or absent. Meditation increases calmness and physical relaxation thus improving psychological balance, coping with illness, and enhancing overall health and well-being. In Western psychology three states of consciousness have been described. However in Eastern philosophy, a fourth state known as the higher state of consciousness has been described. These states of mind are listed in Table 5.1. In the fourth state of mind, incessant thoughts are eliminated and the practitioner experiences a state of deep mental silence. In this state of consciousness, a practitioner feels divine bliss and can be connected with divine consciousness according to *Sutras of Patanjali,* the oldest known text on yoga and meditation. A human soul can be connected to God by achieving a very advanced level of fourth consciousness during meditation which is called *Samadhi.*

The ultimate goal of meditation according to Vedic, Buddhist and Taoist practices is to achieve "*Samadhi,*" a Sanskrit word meaning *a tranquil state of total bliss* also known as "pure awareness," "enlightenment," or "cosmic consciousness." *Samadhi* can be *Savikalpa Samadhi* or *Nirvikalpa Samadhi* where *Savikapla Samadhi* is the initial state of pure bliss and *Nirvikalpa Samadhi* is the ultimate state of bliss where all earthly desires vanish and the human soul is flooded with divine consciousness. However, reaching this state is very difficult for most people. Only highly evolved souls and monks may achieve this state of pure bliss after many years of practice.

This is the state where a person is enlightened or has complete God realization. However, faith in Hinduism or Buddhism is not a prerequisite to practice meditation. Meditation is a non-denominational practice, just like yoga.

Although the goal of meditation is to achieve spiritual bliss, long hours of meditation every day for many years is needed to train the human mind to reach that highest level of consciousness. This is not a realistic goal to achieve for most of us and many practitioners of meditation are not aiming to achieve any state of mind beyond deep relaxation by partially or totally eliminating various thoughts (reducing mental clutter). This reduction or elimination of thought process causes a deep sense of mental calmness and triggers positive emotions ranging from serenity to bliss. With many years of dedicated practice, spiritual growth as well as *Savikalpa Samadhi* can be achieved by some practitioners.

For most of us, meditation is an excellent way to control our minds and release stress from daily life. Practicing meditation for fifteen to twenty minutes once or preferably twice a day has many health benefits. Meditation also causes positive structural and functional changes in the human brain. The top benefits of meditation are summarized in Table 5.2.

Various Types of Meditation

Meditation is a mind-body healing practice where a meditator trains his/her mind to suspend the normal stream of various thoughts. Meditation should be practiced on a regular basis in order to get health benefits. In general a meditator needs to select a quiet place and sit on the floor using a floor mat or even sit comfortably on a chair. There are several approaches including focusing the mind on breathing pattern, focusing on a word or phrase with spiritual meaning (mantra), or focusing on a particular part of the body, feeling sensation of each part in a synchronized manner starting from toes to the head. During meditation one may also focus on a picture and directing his/her love towards an individual. Meditation can be learned from a teacher, a health care professional, or by reading an instructional book or video. Although many types of meditation are practiced today, major meditation techniques practiced in U.S. include:

- Mantra or Sound Meditation: In this type of meditation one may repeat a mantra such as "Om" or during spiritual initiation (Sanskrit: *Diksha*) a teacher may repeat a mantra specific for the student secretly in his/her ear. However, any holy word can be repeated during this type of meditation depending on religious belief.
- Zen Meditation: This type of meditation is practiced by many Buddhist monks. In this meditation both breathing and mind control is practiced and emphasis is on achieving enlightenment through teachings of Buddha.
- Mindfulness-Based Stress Reduction (MBSR) type of Meditation: Dr. Jon Kabat-Zinn in 1979 developed the Mindfulness Based Stress Reduction (MBSR) program at the University of Massachusetts Medical Center. MBSR is an eight week training where participants meet for about ninety minutes once a week and then they can practice this meditation at home. The goal of MBSR practice is to focus attention on moment by moment experiences with an attitude of curiosity, openness, and acceptance. Various practices such as body scanning (paying attention to parts of the body and bodily sensations in sequence starting from feet to the head), breathing (focus on the rise and fall of the abdomen), and even Hatha Yoga may be a part of the MBSR type of meditation. Currently MBSR is offered in over two hundred hospitals in the United States.
- Vipassana Meditation has its roots in ancient Zen meditation practice where a person develops present-moment awareness without being judgmental. This type of meditation has similarity with MBSR, although Vipassana meditation may be linked to Buddhist religious practice where MBSR is a completely secular practice.
- Hatha Yoga: Although this practice is related to the movement of the body through various postures similar to other types of yoga, breathing exercises are also central part of this practice.
- Loving-Kindness Meditation: In this meditation practice, a person during meditation cherishes all living beings on

the earth. This type of meditation is based on Buddhist philosophy but can easily be practiced in a secular way.

- Transcendental Meditation: Taught by Maharishi Mahesh Yogi in the West, where a mantra or a series of mantras is repeated during meditation to achieve mental calmness and eventually a transcendental state of mind similar to the fourth level of consciousness. Usually transcendental meditation is learned from a teacher who may select a mantra specific for the student.

Overall Benefits of Meditation

Regular practice of meditation has many positive effects on both physical health and the mental well-being of a person. Meditation is a very effective way of stress reduction and even as little as fifteen to twenty minutes of meditation a day may be associated with significant stress reduction and a reduced secretion of the stress hormone cortisol. Oxidative stress is associated with pathogenesis of many illness including cardiovascular disease, stroke, diabetes, cancer, obesity, and many others.[1] Meditation also reduces blood pressure, improves immune functions, and is effective in reducing pain. Physical health benefits of meditation are summarized in Table 5.3.

Meditation increases positive emotion and mood by reducing anxiety. Meditation is an excellent way to avoid depression and other mental illness. Meditation may also be useful in overcoming substance abuse. Long term practice of meditation alters brain structure in a very positive way. Moreover, meditation is also associated with slower brain waves including theta waves that may be related to transcendental spiritual experience associated with long term practice of meditation. Major mental health benefits of meditation are summarized in Table 5.4.

Meditation, Stress Relief, and Reduced Oxidative Stress

Stress in classical term indicates a situation where a human has to decide between fight or flight. Stress is an adaptive mechanism of humans and animals alike in response to external threats. It is a complex defense mechanism to protect the body. Psychological stress is a part of human life, but prolonged exposure to stress increases free radical production of the body and also reduces antioxidant defense. As a result a person experiencing chronic stress is also under increased oxidative stress. Chronic exposure to increased oxidative stress is linked to many illnesses. Prolonged stress may also cause depression. Experiments with the healthy human population indicated a link between stress and cardiovascular diseases. Stress can contribute to initiation and even progression of certain types of cancer. Stress also weakens immune function.[2] Various symptoms of stress are listed in Table 5.5. Various results of chronic stress are listed in Table 5.6.

Stress induces a complex biological process first in the human brain, which causes secretion of various stress related molecules that affect virtually all organs. Stress induces the hypothalamic-pituitary-adrenal axis of the human brain and as a result of this activation, adrenal glands secrete glucocorticoids which are known as "stress hormones." Cortisol, a steroid, is the primary glucocorticoid hormone found in humans although modest levels of cortisol are present in human blood and the concentration varies with the time of day (cortisol concentration is lowest at night and highest in the morning). Cortisol increases blood pressure and blood sugar while decreasing immune function. Cortisol also increases oxidative stress and can cause damage to nerve cells (neurons) and may reduce concentrations of antioxidant enzymes.[3]

Meditation can reduce stress as well as oxidative stress. Therefore, many health benefits of meditation are due to the ability of this mind-body practice to reduce stress of everyday life. Sharma and Rush reviewed seventeen published studies dealing with the stress reduction capacity of the MBSR type of meditation in healthy individuals. The authors reported that sixteen out of seventeen studies demonstrated positive outcomes related to the reduction of stress and anxiety. The authors concluded that the MBSR type of meditation is an effective approach towards stress management in healthy individuals.[4] Goyal et al. reviewed forty-seven clinical trials involving 3,515 participants and concluded that the practice of meditation is associated with stress reduction. Moreover, eight weeks of meditation can effectively reduce anxiety, depression and perception of pain.[5]

Transcendental meditation is very effective in reducing stress. Elder et al. studied the effectiveness of transcendental meditation in reducing stress, depression, and burnout in teachers involved in teaching students with severe behavioral problems. According to this study, approximately 70% of teachers are under frequent stress related to student discipline issues, which may eventually result in burnout. Burnout is a syndrome associated with emotional exhaustion, negative attitude towards others, and dissatisfaction with one's job performance. The authors recruited 40 secondary school teachers and support staff of a residential school and divided them into two groups. One group was taught transcendental meditation by certified teachers and was instructed to practice meditation fifteen to twenty minutes twice a day at home. The other subjects (control group) did not practice transcendental meditation. After four months, teachers who practiced transcendental meditation showed significantly reduced perception of stress, depression, and burnout phenomenon compared to the control group. The authors concluded that practice of transcendental meditation for four months was very effective in reducing psychological distress in teachers and support staffs working in a residential therapeutic school for students with sever behavioral problems.[6]

Loving-Kindness Meditation is also very effective in reducing stress. In this type of practice, a practitioner first directs love to himself or herself—we often do not love ourselves enough—and then to a close friend or a family member or a spiritual teacher who has contributed significantly to the practitioner's life. Finally, the practitioner can love all living beings, even an individual who the practitioner hates. Kemper et al. studied seven inexperienced and five experienced healthy meditators in one sitting who participated in a twenty minute loving-kindness meditation. The authors observed significant stress reduction after meditation even in inexperienced meditators. However, experienced meditators had significantly lower stress and lower heart rate before meditation compared to inexperienced meditators. As expected, stress levels were more significantly reduced after meditation in experienced meditators.[7] Based on the review of medical literature, Hoffman concluded that loving-kindness meditation is effective in reducing depression, social anxiety, marital conflict, anger, and coping with long-term caregiving.[8]

The silent repetition of a word or a phrase (mantra) with spiritual significance is an ancient form of meditative prayer and is very effective in reducing stress. A mantra can be repeated anytime of a day and also in response to stress. Common mantras are listed in Table 5.7. Based on a study using sixty-two outpatient veterans, Borman et al. concluded that mantra repetition significantly reduced stress and anxiety in the subjects and also improved quality of life and spiritual well-being.[9] In another study by the same author, thirty veterans (97% male) and thirty-six hospital employees (86% female) with mean age of fifty-six years participated in a five-week study involving mantra repetition. Each subject selected his or her own mantra based on religious belief, but each mantra had spiritual significance. The authors received responses from fifty-five participants who identified 147 incidents where mantra repetition was helpful. These incidents included managing emotions other than stress (51%), stress (23.8%), insomnia (12.9%), and unwanted thoughts (12.3%). The authors concluded that mantra repetition is useful in reducing stress and improving mental and spiritual well-being. The authors also mentioned other studies that demonstrated lowering blood pressure, lowering stress and lowering anger following short term practice of mantra repetition. Long term effects include improving mood, lowering pain, lowering depression and lowering frequency of insomnia.[10]

Meditation Lowers Serum Cortisol

Cortisol is the main stress hormone secreted in response to stress. High blood cortisol in response to chronic stress has many adverse health effects. Meditation is an effective method of reducing cortisol level in blood (serum cortisol). In one study using thirty second-year medical students, Turakitwanakan et al. demonstrated that after four days of mindfulness meditation, the average cortisol level reduced from the pre-meditation level of 381.93 nmol/L (13.8 mg/dL) to 306.39 nmol/L collected after four days of meditation. These readings were all collected at 8 a.m., and levels usually only range 5-23 mg/dL. The reduction of cortisol levels (19.7%) in these subjects was statistically significant.[11]

Brand et al. studied serum cortisol levels in nine experienced meditators and eleven novices. However, novices underwent eight-week training of MBSR. For experienced meditators, morning serum cortisol decreased with length of experience (serum cortisol is higher in the morning and lower at night). For novices, serum cortisol levels also decreased from pre-training level after eight weeks of MBSR training. Moreover, sleep quality was improved in novices after receiving MBSR training.[12]

In another report, the authors studied whether the practice of transcendental meditation may reduce the cortisol response to a metabolic challenge. In this study, the authors compared-post challenge cortisol level (after ingestion of 75 grams glucose orally) in 16 women who were long-term practitioners of transcendental meditation and fourteen women who did not meditate. After ingestion of glucose, salivary cortisol levels were significantly higher in women who did not meditate than in women who had practiced meditation for a long time. Since glucose increases cortisol secretion, the authors concluded that lower cortisol response to a metabolic challenge in women who practiced meditation indicated improved endocrine regulation and disease preventing capability of transcendental meditation.[13]

Meditation Improves the Antioxidant Status of the Body

A lowered cortisol level is one of the ways by which meditation reduces stress level. Free radicals are produced during normal cellular metabolism. These free radicals include superoxide radicals, hydrogen peroxide, and extremely reactive hydroxyl radicals. Free radicals damage lipid molecules, and malondialdehyde, an end product of lipid peroxidation, is commonly measured as a marker of oxidative stress. The practice of meditation is associated with lower oxidative stress and higher levels of antioxidant enzymes in blood. Lowering oxidative stress may be a common mechanism by which meditation reduces risk of various diseases that are associated with increased oxidative stress.

Long term transcendental and Zen meditators usually show diminished oxidative stress as evidenced by reduced lipid peroxidation products in blood. Moreover, the practice of meditation also increases serum glutathione level (a potent antioxidant) and activities of several antioxidant enzymes, including catalase, superoxide dismutase, glutathione peroxidase, and glutathione reductase.[14] Kim et al. studied twenty subjects who practiced Zen meditation and twenty control subjects who did not meditate and found significantly lower serum levels of malondialdehyde in meditators compared non-meditations. This indicates less oxidative stress. The authors concluded that Zen meditation can reduce oxidative stress.[15]

Meditation Reduces Hospital Admission and Doctor's Office Visits

The practice of transcendental meditation for fifteen to twenty minutes twice a day on a regular basis is associated with good health, as evidenced by a lower rate of hospitalization and a lower rate of doctor's office visits among meditators compared to non-meditators. Orme-Johnson studied five years' worth of the medical insurance utilization statistics of approximately 2,000 regular participants of transcendental meditation and 600,000 members of the same insurance carrier (control group). The author observed that meditators had lower medical utilization rates compared to the control group. In the age group of 40 years and up, people who meditated had 73.7% fewer outpatient visits compared to non-meditators. In addition, meditators had 53.3% fewer hospital admissions than people who did not meditate. Interestingly, admission to hospitals per 1000 people were 87% lower in meditators admitted for heart diseases, 87.3% lower for nervous system diseases, 55.4% lower for benign and malignant tumors, 30.4% lower for infectious diseases and 30.6% lower for psychiatric illnesses.[16] This study also indicates that meditation is very effective in reducing the risk of heart diseases, nervous system diseases, cancer, infectious diseases, and psychiatric illnesses.

Herron studied the highest-spending Quebec health insurance enrollees (1,418 subjects) who practiced transcendental meditation and people who did not meditate (1,418 subjects). The Quebec government health agency provided the total physician payments in both groups. Before starting meditation, the yearly payments to physicians did not change between these two groups. However, after one year of practice of transcendental meditation, physician payments in transcendental meditation group declined by 11% and after five years declined by 28% compared to people who did not practice meditation.[17]

Meditation Reduces Risk of Cardiovascular Disease and Stroke

Meditation is an effective way to reduce the risk of many cardiovascular diseases, including myocardial infarction and heart failure. Meditation is an excellent way of reducing stress that results in normalization of neuroendocrine system and reduces oxidative stress. Increased oxidative stress is a risk factor for cardiovascular diseases. Meditation also improves lipid profile in blood and this favorable lipid profile (reduced levels of cholesterol, triglycerides, and low density lipoprotein cholesterol, also known as bad cholesterol, as well as increased levels of high density lipoprotein cholesterol, known as good cholesterol) also the lowers risk of heart diseases. In addition, meditation is effective in lowering blood pressure which has a positive impact on heart function.

Atherosclerosis is process by which arterial walls supplying blood to the heart are thickened due to buildup of fats, cholesterol and other substances (plaques). As a result, blood supply in the heart is restricted. Sometimes such plaque may burst and a blood clot may develop, thus stopping or restricting the flow of blood in the heart. This phenomenon is known as a myocardial infarction, also known as a heart attack. Walton et al. reviewed papers published in the field of effects of transcendental meditation on cardiac health and commented that the practice of transcendental meditation alone for one year reduces the likelihood of heart attack or stroke by 33%. In addition, the practice of transcendental meditation is also associated with a reduction in atherosclerotic plaque both in inner-city blacks with hypertension and in older white Americans. Walton further commented that lower lipid peroxide levels were observed in subjects practicing transcendental meditation, indicating lower oxidative stress. A significant reduction in serum cholesterol after 11 months of practicing transcendental meditation has also been reported.[18] In another report, Koika et al. concluded that all types of meditation are associated with blood pressure control, a reduction in lipid peroxidation (reduced oxidative stress), and a reduction of cellular senescence. All such mechanisms contribute to better cardiovascular health. Therefore, all types of meditations are effective in reducing risk of heart diseases.[19]

Meditation Reduces Risk of Cancer

Meditation is effective in improving physical and mental health of cancer survivors. Meditation is also effective in pain control among cancer patients. In addition, some investigators observed that meditation may reduce relapses or slow the progress of certain types of cancer. Dobos et al., based on a study of 117 cancer survivors who practiced meditation, observed reduced cancer-related symptoms, including fatigue, pain, insomnia, constipation, anxiety, and depression. The authors concluded that meditation is an effective way of improving physical and mental health of cancer survivors.[20]

Robb et al., based on a study using teachers who teach meditation, showed that long-term meditation is associated with lower incidences of cancer. The authors commented that stress reduction and reduced oxidative stress in meditation teachers may be responsible for lowering the risk of cancer in these subjects.[21]

Meditation Reduces Blood Pressure and Improves Blood Glucose Control in Diabetic Patients

Diabetes is a risk factor for cardiovascular diseases. Moreover, many diabetic patients also suffer from high blood pressure. Regular meditation may be very helpful for controlling both blood pressure and blood sugar when paired with medications, diet, and exercise in diabetic patients. Anderson et al., based on review and analysis of nine clinical trials published in medical literatures, concluded that transcendental meditation may reduce systolic and diastolic blood pressures by approximately 4.7 and 3.3 mm of Hg respectively. The authors commented that such reductions in blood pressure are clinically significant.[22]

A mindfulness-based stress reduction (MBSR) meditation program is associated with better control of blood sugar in diabetes patients as reflected by lower hemoglobin A1c (HbA1c, also called glycosylated hemoglobin, is a marker of blood sugar control over a four-month period). Using eleven adult patients with Type 2 Diabetes (non-insulin dependent diabetes that can be controlled by oral medication, diet, and exercise) who participated in one month MBSR program, Rosenzweig et al. showed that mean HbA1c was reduced by 0.48%, a significant reduction in these patients. Moreover, reduced anxiety, depression, and psychological stress were also observed in these patients.[23] In another study involving 50 patients who participated in seating-breathing type meditation for three weeks, Chaiopanont et al. showed an average reduction of postprandial blood glucose (blood glucose two hours after meal) by 19.26 mg/dL. Diastolic blood pressure was also reduced by 3.05 mm Hg.[24]

Meditation and the Immune System

Strenuous exercise may suppress the immune system. However, Solberg et al., based on a study using six meditating and six non-meditating male runners for a period of six months, reported that meditation is effective in modifying the suppressive effect of strenuous exercise on the immune system.[25] Morgan et al., based on a review of thirty-four studies and meta-analysis, concluded that seven to sixteen weeks of meditation reduced the level of interleukin-6 and of C-reactive protein in blood, indicating that meditation reduces markers of inflammation.[26]

Meditation Reduces Chronic Pain

Meditation is effective in reducing chronic pain. Chronic tension headache is the most common type of headache. In one study, Kiran et al. divided fifty patients with chronic tension headaches into two groups. One group of thirty patients received eight lessons of meditation (known as Raja-Yoga meditation) for relaxation in addition to medications (analgesics and muscle relaxants) while the twenty patients in the second group received medications only. After eight weeks, 94% of the patients in Group 1 reported highly significant relief of headache while only 36% of patients in Group 2 reported highly significant pain relief. Moreover, the duration and frequency of the headaches were also reduced by 91% and 97% in patients in Group 1 compared to 36% and 49% reductions in Group 2 patients who did not meditate. The authors concluded that meditation is highly effective in reducing intensity of pain, duration, and frequency of tension headaches in patients suffering from such headaches.[27]

In another study, Wells et al. divided nineteen patients suffering from migraines into two groups. One group of ten patients practiced MBSR meditation while another group of nine patients received standard care. The authors observed that patients who practiced MBSR had fewer migraines per month compared to patients who did not participate in meditation. Moreover, the intensity of migraines was less severe in patients who participated in meditation compared to patients who did not meditate.[28]

Reiner et al., based on review of sixteen studies, concluded that MBSR meditation significantly decreases the intensity of pain in patients suffering from chronic pain.[29] Another study involved 109 patients with chronic pain who were divided into two groups with one group practicing MBSR meditation while the other group did not meditate, Ia Cour et al., based on a two and a half year follow-up, concluded that MBSR contributes positively to pain management and can exert clinically relevant effects in patients suffering from chronic pain.[30] Morone et al., using twenty-seven adult patients over sixty-five years old who all suffered from chronic back pain, reported that MBSR meditation was effective in reducing back pain. In addition, these older adults also reported better sleep quality, enhanced well-being and overall improvement in quality of life.[31]

Meditation Improves Sleep Quality and Reduces Symptoms of Insomnia

Sleep disturbances are common among the elderly population. In one study, the authors divided forty-nine older adults (mean age 66.4 years) with moderate sleep disturbances into two groups. One group of twenty-seven older adults practiced MBSR meditation while the other group of twenty-four older adults received sleep hygiene education. Older adults who participated in meditation showed better sleep quality, lesser incidence of insomnia, lesser fatigue, and lesser depression compared to older adults who received sleep hygiene education only. The authors concluded that MBSR meditation may improve sleep quality and lower daytime impairment among older adults with sleep disturbances.[32]

Ong et al., based on a study using fifty-four patients with chronic insomnia, observed that patients who practiced MBSR had better sleep quality and lesser symptoms of insomnia in a six month follow-up. The authors concluded that MBSR is a viable treatment option for adults with chronic insomnia.[33] Even self-relaxation techniques may improve sleep quality and cognitive function compared to sleep hygiene education. Sun et al., using eighty older patients and a one-year follow-up, showed that self-relaxation techniques have a significant positive effect on sleep quality and cognitive function compared to sleep hygiene education.[34]

Meditation Increases Overall Longevity and Reverses Aging

Reduction of gray matter within the hippocampal region of the brain is a normal manifestation of aging. Kurth et al., using fifty long-term meditators and fifty control subjects, showed through high resolution magnetic resonance imaging (MRI) that there was less age-related degeneration in meditators compared to subjects who did not meditate.[35] Inside the nucleus of a cell, human genes are arranged along twisted, double-stranded molecules of DNA called chromosomes. Stretches of DNA at the ends of the chromosomes are known as telomeres, which get shorter as cells divide. When telomeres get too short, cells cannot divide anymore and die. This shortening of telomeres is associated with aging and may indicate decreased longevity, while longer telomeres indicate decreased aging and increased longevity. Hoge et al., based on a study using fifteen women who practiced loving-kindness meditation and twenty-two women who did not meditate but were matched for age, showed that loving kindness meditation was associated with longer relative telomere length in meditators compared to non-meditators. Interestingly, women who meditated had lower body mass index than non-meditators. The authors concluded that meditation practice may increase relative telomere length, which is a biomarker of increased longevity.[36]

Alexander et al. studied the effects of transcendental meditation on longevity using seventy-three residents of eight homes with mean age of eighty-one years. The authors randomly assigned these subjects into three groups, where subjects in one group practiced transcendental meditation, subjects in a second group received mindfulness meditation training, and subjects in a third group did not participate in any kind of meditation. After three years of follow-up, survival rate was 100% in subjects who practiced transcendental meditation and 87.5% in people who practiced mindfulness meditation in contrast to a low survival rate among elderly who did not meditation. The authors concluded that meditation may increase longevity.[37]

Meditation Improves the Brain's Function

Many studies indicate that meditation improves cognitive function, the processing of information, concentration, and memory. Meditation reduces cortisol secretion, and as a result, the level of brain-derived neurotrophic factor (which enhances growth and survival of neurons) is increased. Meditation also reduces oxidative stress, and as a result, age-related neurodegeneration is reduced. Neuroprotective effects of meditation are validated by the study of brain waves (monitored by electroencephalogram, or EEG) and imaging studies. In general, meditation enhances cognitive function and brain plasticity. Enhancement of brain plasticity results in better neuronal connectivity which improves memory, concentration, and other functions of the brain.[38]

Luders et al. compared brain images from fifty adult meditators and fifty adult non-meditators. Results demonstrated that people who practiced meditation for many years had more folds in the cortical structure (gyrification) of the brain. Such changes are associated with increased capacity of the brain to process information, and as a result, mental focus and intelligence is increased.[39] Holzel et al. commented that gyrification is reduced with aging. Therefore, increased gyrification in meditators also indicates that meditation may slow and even stall normal aging of the brain. Meditation also increases gray matter in certain areas of the brain, including the left hippocampus, posterior cingulate cortex, temporoparietal junction, and cerebellum. These regions of the brain are involved in learning, memory, and emotional regulations.[40] Meditation also increases white matter in the brain, which may be related to theta waves generated during meditation. Theta waves produce a molecular cascade that increases myelin and improves neuronal connectivity. As a result, the mental capacity of the brain is improved.[41] Specific changes in the brain due to practice of meditation are listed in Table 5.8.

The prefrontal cortex of the brain plays an important role in controlling cognitive behavior, personality, decision-making, and social behavior. Expert meditators show activation of the prefrontal cortex and have better judgment, more concentration, and a better ability to differentiate between conflicting thoughts than non-meditators. Meditators also show thicker cortex in the pre-frontal cortex and temporal regions of the brain. As a result, meditators have better cognitive functions than non-meditators. Meditation also activates the hippocampus, amygdala, and anterior cingulate regions of the brain, which are responsible for motivation, memory, and emotion. Moreover, meditation also increases bridging between the left hemisphere and right hemisphere of the brain (through the corpus callosum), thus enhancing mental strength. Meditation increases levels of gamma-aminobutyric acid, a neurotransmitter which reduces anxiety and depression. In addition, the predominance of the parasympathetic nervous system during meditation decreases heart rate, blood pressure, and the consumption of oxygen. Moreover, meditation increases melatonin production by the pineal gland of the brain, which contributes to good night sleep, mental calmness, and decreased awareness of pain.[42]

Meditation Reduces Depression and Degenerative Psychiatric Illness

As mentioned earlier, meditation is an effective method for reducing depression and anxiety. Miller et al., based on a study of twenty-four depressed patients who practiced meditation for six weeks, observed that meditation was effective in reducing the symptoms of depression and improving spiritual growth and mental health among depressed patients.[43] In another study using 322 adults who participated in an eight-week, community-based MBSR program, Greeson et al. observed that adults who participated in the MBSR program showed significant reduction in depressive symptoms compared to controls and such reduction in depression was not associated with religious affiliation, gender or age. The authors concluded that MBSR-based meditation is an effective method of reducing depression.[44]

Posttraumatic stress disorder is a serious psychological issue that often affects veterans. In one study, the Kearney et al. reported that loving-kindness meditation is very effective in reducing symptoms of posttraumatic stress disorder among veterans[45].

Psychiatric illness is common among prisoners. Himelstein reviewed reports dealing with the effect of meditation programs on prisoners and concluded that meditation-based programs in prisons provide an enhancement of psychological well-being, a decrease in substance abuse, and a decreased likelihood of recidivism.[46]

Age-related dementia and cognitive decline are sometimes associated with advanced age. Meditation can be considered a non-pharmacological intervention aimed at the prevention of cognitive decline in elderly. Meditation is very effective in reducing the aging process of the brain, as Luders reported that the average cortical thickness of a forty- to fifty-year-old meditation practitioner was similar to a twenty- to thirty-year-old control subject.[47] Therefore, the regular practice of meditation is effective in slowing the rate of neural degeneration. Neural degeneration (neurodegeneration or brain degeneration) is related to many psychiatric illnesses, including age-related dementia, Alzheimer's disease, Parkinson's disease, and Huntington's disease. Therefore, meditation may slow, stall, or even reverse age-related brain degeneration and as a result reduces the risk of developing diseases related to increased brain degeneration. In general, after the age of forty, the human brain decreases by volume and weight at a rate of approximately 5% every decade, and as a result, the elderly population is more vulnerable to diseases related to brain degeneration. Meditation has a brain-preserving effect, thus reducing risks of developing neurodegenerative diseases.[47]

Meditation Reduces Addiction to Nicotine, Alcohol, and Drugs

More than five million deaths per year are attributed to tobacco smoking. Nicotine, found in tobacco, is responsible for smoking addictions. However, meditation is beneficial in reducing smoking habits. Tank et al. reported that two weeks of meditation training (five hours total) was associated with a 60% reduction in smoking among subjects who meditated but no such reduction was observed in people who received only relaxation training. The authors concluded that meditation improves self-control capacity and reduces smoking.[48]

Shafil et al. surveyed the frequency of alcohol use in 126 individuals identified as practitioners of transcendental meditation and matched a control group consisting of ninety individuals who did not report any meditation. No individuals in the control group discontinued drinking beer or wine over a two-year period, but 40% of the subjects who practiced meditation discontinued alcohol within the first six months, and after twenty-five to thirty-nine months of meditation, 60% of the individuals who meditated discontinued alcohol consumption altogether. In addition, 54% of the individuals who meditated discontinued use of hard liquors while only 1% of the non-meditating individuals discontinued the use of hard liquor. The authors concluded that meditation could be an effective tool in preventing alcohol abuse.[49]

MBSR meditation is very effective in preventing substance abuse. Black, based on reviews of over twenty-five papers, commented that MBSR and other types of meditation are effective adjunct therapies in substance abusers to reduce or prevent the future tendency of substance abuse.[50] Aron et al. reviewed papers dealing with effect of transcendental meditation in reducing addiction and commented that four to twelve weeks of transcendental meditation caused significant decline in alcohol, tobacco, and marijuana use among college students. Therefore, transcendental meditation is very effective in preventing alcohol and drug abuse.[51]

Qigong meditation blends relaxation, breathing, guided imagery, inward attention, and mindfulness to achieve a tranquil state of mind. Chen et al. studied the effects of Qigong meditation using 248 subjects who were enrolled in a residential drug rehabilitation program. Participants selected to meditate or receive stress management and relaxation training. After four weeks, 92% of the subjects in the meditation group successfully completed drug rehabilitation program while 78% of the subjects in the stress management group successfully completed the program. Interestingly, meditative therapy was more effective in female substance abusers than in male substance abusers. The authors concluded that meditative therapy is useful in preventing substance abuse.[52]

Meditation Reduces Eating Disorders and Obesity

Meditation is effective in controlling binge eating and emotional eating resulting in weight loss. Kristeller et al., using eighteen obese women with eating disorders who participated in a six-week meditation-based group intervention program, reported that binge eating frequency reduced from 4.02/week to 1.57/week after meditation training. The authors concluded that meditation is an effective tool in controlling binge eating in obese women.[53] In another report, the authors reviewed fourteen studies dealing with the effects of meditation on binge eating, emotional eating and weight loss. The authors concluded that meditation is effective in reducing binge eating, emotional eating, and may aid in weight loss.[54]

Meditation and Spiritual Bliss

During a religious or spiritual experience, certain areas of the brain are activated. Moreover, neurotransmitters such as dopamine and serotonin also play important role when an individual experiences religious or spiritual bless (see Chapter 3). Most people practice meditation for stress reduction and to achieve a tranquil state of mind. However, the goal of certain types of meditations, such as transcendental meditation or Buddhist Zen meditation, is to achieve a fourth state of consciousness known as thoughtful awareness or cosmic consciousness. This fourth state of consciousness is also called *Turiya Chetana* in Sanskrit, indicating that in this state of mind, a meditator directly feels divine bliss and is enlightened. The fourth and highest stage, known as *Nirvikalpa Samadhi* is the ultimate state of consciousness when a human soul is flooded with divine consciousness.

Some investigators studied EEG patterns in subjects while meditating. These subjects ranged from new practitioners to Buddhist monks with many years of practice in meditation. Lagopoulos et al. examined the EEG profiles of participants who participated in Acem meditation, a nondirective meditation technique, for twenty minutes and then twenty minutes of relaxation with eyes closed. There was a fifteen minute break in between the two sessions. The authors observed that during meditation, theta waves were more abundant in the frontal and temporal central region of the brain. Theta waves represent a very relaxed state of mind where attention is focused into the inner self. Theta waves also unlock the door to the unconscious mind and may be related to experiences of spiritual bliss during meditation. In addition, authors also observed significantly greater alpha waves in the posterior of the brain compared to the frontal part. Alpha waves are slow frequency waves associated with a relaxed state of mind.[55] Recently, Pasquini et al., based on a study of seventeen Buddhist monks and fourteen controls, showed that the frequency of weekly meditation was associated with increased theta waves in the EEG.[56] Mindfulness based meditation also increases theta waves (6-8 Hz) in the frontal part of the brain.

Tsai studied EEG activities in long-term meditators at rest, during breathing meditation, and when an advanced meditative state was reached. During breathing meditation, significantly higher bilateral theta waves (comparable activity in the left and right hemispheres of the brain) were recorded than during the resting stage. However, during the advanced state of meditation, both increased theta and alpha waves were observed on both the left and right sides of the brain. The authors concluded that internalized attention during meditation was reflected as theta waves, which were enhanced as meditators progressed to advanced state of meditation.[57]

Travis commented that during transcendental meditation, higher frontal alpha-1 waves (8-10 Hz) are observed along with higher parasympathetic activity and a lower breathing rate. Cosmic consciousness experienced by long term practitioners of transcendental meditation is due to alpha-1 waves along with delta waves, higher brain integration, greater emotional stability and decreased anxiety during challenging tasks.[58] Mason et al. observed no difference in delta waves (characteristics of deep sleep) between long term practitioners of transcendental meditation and controls.[59] Interestingly, Lutz et al. observed high frequency gamma waves (25-42 Hz) along with low frequency theta and alpha waves (4-13 Hz) in Buddhist monks with many years of meditation experience. This gamma band may be related to many years of mental training involved with the temporal integrative mechanism and neural changes, because during gamma wave activity higher mental functions can be performed.[60]

Neurotransmitters may also play important roles in the experience of spiritual bliss during meditation. Serotonin is an important neurotransmitter which controls mood, behavior, and appetite. Increased levels of serotonin are associated with mood elevation while decreased level may cause depression. Selective serotonin reuptake inhibitors (SSRIs), which are capable of increasing serotonin levels in the brain, are used in treating depression. Increased concentrations of serotonin metabolites are observed in urine of meditators, indicating that meditation may increase brain serotonin levels. Dopamine, the neurotransmitter associated with the reward system of the brain, is also increased during meditation.[61]

Conclusion

The regular practice of any type of meditation can offer many health benefits. Meditation is very effective in reducing stress and the many benefits of meditation are directly attributable to stress reduction. Moreover, during meditation, the activity of the parasympathetic nervous system is increased and as a result, blood pressure, respiratory rate, and heart rate are decreased. In addition, the release of stress hormones, such as cortisol, is also reduced. Meditation stimulates the release of natural opiates of the brain, known as endorphins, which have a calming effect on the brain. Meditation also increases mental focus, memory, cognition, and helps to achieve a higher level of emotional balance. Meditation slows down the aging process of the brain, thus reducing the risk of developing age-related dementia and other neurodegenerative diseases. The ultimate goal of meditation is to achieve spiritual enlightenment and cosmic consciousness. Even though most of us may not be able to reach such a high state of mind, many physical and mental health benefits of meditation can be achieved by practicing meditation for fifteen to twenty minutes per day.

Table 5.1 Various states of consciousness in Western psychology and Eastern philosophy

Western Psychology	Eastern Philosophy
• Sleep • Dream • Wakefulness	• Sleep • Dream • Wakefulness • Thoughtless awareness or cosmic consciousness

Table 5.2 Top benefits of meditation

- Benefits at the physical level: stress relief and feeling of deep relaxation. As a result, oxidative stress in the body is reduced, which translates into better health and a longer life.
- Individuals who practice meditation have much lower incidences of doctor's office visits and hospitalization compared to people who do not meditate.
- Benefits at the cognitive level: improved mental focus, memory, self-control, and better ability to remain calm in the face of stress
- Benefits at the emotional level: happier life due to positive mood, emotional stability, and the capacity to cope with negative life events
- Prevents depression and reduces incidence of psychiatric illness
- Prevents or delays onset of degenerative mental illnesses such as Alzheimer's disease and Parkinson's disease
- Reduces aging process and increases longevity

Table 5.3 Physical health benefits of meditation

- Reduces stress, and as a result, antioxidant capacity of blood is increased
- People who practice meditation have fewer hospital admissions and fewer doctor's office visits
- Slows down the aging process and increases longevity
- Effective in reducing the incidence of cardiovascular diseases, including heart attack and stroke
- Can reduce incidences of certain types of cancers
- Effective in lowering blood pressure, but hypertensive people also may need medication
- Can lower blood sugar along with medication
- Boosts immune system
- Effective method for reducing chronic pain
- Improves sleep quality and reduces symptoms of insomnia

Table 5.4 Mental health benefits of meditation

- Improves brain's structure and function
- Shifts activity of the prefrontal cortex from right to left hemisphere of the brain and such shifts makes a person more enthusiastic, calmer and happier
- Effective in improving mental focus and concentration
- Meditators are less vulnerable to stresses and better at regulating immediate responses to negative stimuli than people who do not meditate
- Regular meditation can delay or prevent degenerative mental disorders such as Alzheimer's disease, Parkinson's disease, and Huntington disease
- Reduces addiction to nicotine, alcohol, and drugs
- Can help with eating disorders
- Can help with spiritual growth

Table 5.5 Signs and symptoms of stress

Short term stress	Chronic stress
• Increased blood pressure • Increased heart rate • Tension headache • Anxiety attack • Back pain • Diarrhea • Upset stomach	• Unhealthy eating pattern causing either weight gain or weight loss • Trouble sleeping, or insomnia • Fatigue • Problems with mental health • May have difficulty with marriage or relationship • Onset of depression

Table 5.6 Results of chronic stress*

- Increased risk of cardiovascular diseases including myocardial infarction (heart attack) and heart failure
- Increased risk of cancer
- Weakened immune system
- Inflammation
- Increased risk of diabetes
- High blood pressure (hypertension)
- Increased risk of migraine headache
- Increased risk of asthma
- Increased risk of obesity
- Gastric acidity
- Premature aging and reduced life span
- Increased risk of developing degenerative mental disorders, such as age-related dementia or Alzheimer's disease

*Most of these illnesses are related to chronic exposure to excessive oxidative stress

Table 5.7 Some common mantras

Hindu

- Om
- Om Shanti (Peace be everywhere)
- Sohum (I am also God)
- Om Namah Shivaya (Adoration to Lord Shiva)
- Ram Ram Sri Ram (Ram is a mythological person of epic Ramayana)

Christian

- Jesus or Lord Jesus Christ
- My God and my all
- Hail Mary or Ava Maria

Buddhist

- Om Mani Padme Hum (An invocation of self)

Islam

- Allah (God almighty)
- Bismallah

Table 5.8 Specific changes in the brain due to practice of meditation

Specific changes in the brain	Comments
Cortical gyrification	Gyrification refers to the increased cortical folding in the brain that increases mental capacity. Cortical folding is the reason why the human brain has a wrinkled appearance.
Experienced meditators show thicker cortex in pre-frontal cortex and temporal region of the brain	A thicker cortex is associated with improved mental capacity. Thickness of the cortex reduces with advanced age. Therefore, meditation may prevent the brain from age-related degeneration.
Increased gray matter (in left hippocampus, posterior cingulate cortex, left temporal junction, and cerebellum)	An increase in gray matter in these regions of the brain may positively impact learning process, memory, emotional balance, self-referential processing and perspective taking.
Increased efficiency of white matter	Theta brain waves induced by meditation may produce a molecular cascade that increases myelin and improves the connectivity of the brain. As result, overall mental capacity is increased.

Table 5.8 cont.

Specific changes in the brain	Comments
Increased brain plasticity	Brain plasticity improves neural connections in the brain, thus increasing mental capacity.
Reduces age-related brain degeneration	An MRI study showed lesser age-related degeneration in meditators compared to subjects who did not meditate

Chapter 6
The Science of Prayer and Complementary Healing Modalities

Introduction

The word "prayer" is derived from the Latin word *precari* meaning begging. Prayer is an integral part of all religions and is the most ancient form of communication with divine. Prayer is also used in various non-denominational religious or spiritual practices. Many religions have set prayers for specific occasions. For example, the Lord's Prayer in Christianity or the Gayatri mantra in Hinduism. Rig-Veda, the ancient Holy Text of Hinduism, originated approximately 5,000 years ago and is full of hymns praising thirty-three different gods and goddesses. Devotional songs praising Gods are also a form of prayer. However, prayers serve as heart to heart communication between a faithful and God, where a faithful may use his or her own language to communicate with God without using any religious text. Prayers can also be conducted in silence. Chanting religious or Holy Text phrases during meditation can also be considered a form of prayer. In Christianity, prayer can be a petition to God for help with daily life, recovery from illness, or developing a more personal relationship with God. A prayer can also be for someone else (intercessory prayer).

A person who prays hopes that God or a Supreme Being is listening to our petitions and has the power to grant such petitions even if it violates a natural law. For example, one may pray for a person to recover from a terminal illness although such a thing is not medically feasible. Although prayers may be used to ask God for a favor or fulfill a wish, prayers are most commonly made for the healing of oneself or someone closely related when standard medical care fails to produce desired results. Sometimes, prayers are the last resort for family members of a dying patient, and they often hope for miracles. Medical miracles are discussed in the bonus section with emphasis on specific case reports. In this chapter, scientific research showing effects of prayers on healing is discussed. In the opinion of this author, medical literature on the effectiveness of prayer is full of controversies with some studies reporting a positive outcome while other studies report no correlation between prayer and medical outcome.

There are various distant healings and touch based healings. Touch based healings may be Reiki, or healing touch. Distant healing may also include distant Reiki. Although some of the touch based and distant healings are not religious in nature, most healers have some belief in the existence of a higher being. A healer may believe that she or he is capable of tapping energy from the universe's energy and is capable of using such energy for healing.

Prevalence of Prayer

Prayer is a very common practice in U.S. According to a Gallup poll, 95% of Americans believe in the existence of God and 82% of Americans believe in the healing power of personal prayer. Moreover, 77% of Americans believe that God can cure a serious illness. In addition, 94% of patients admitted to the hospital believe that spiritual health is as important as physical health and 77% believe that physicians should consider a patient's spiritual needs as a part of their medical care.[1]

Saudi et al. reported that 96% of patients pray one day before cardiac surgery to deal with the stress and 97% reported that prayer was helpful.[2] In a study based on 493 patients in a cancer hospital in Texas, Richardson et al. reported that 79.2% patients prayed for their own health and 71.9% said that someone else prayed for them.[3] When people face illness, especially chronic illness, they tend to become more religious or spiritual and have increased belief in prayer. Prayers are not only practiced by individuals who participate in organized religions but also by people who participate in non-denominational spiritual practices. If prayer is considered a complementary medicine due to its healing effect, then compared to Reiki, yoga, or meditation, prayer is the most common form of complementary medicine.

Jors et al. classified health-related prayers into five categories, including disease-centered prayer, assurance-centered prayer, God-centered prayer, other-centered prayer, and lamentations.[4] The characteristics of various categories of prayers are summarized in Table 6.1. From a scientific standpoint, intercessory prayers are the best suited for investigation because patients can be randomly assigned to either receive or not to receive intercessory prayer, but as expected, all patients receive usual medical care. Moreover, patients may be blinded to whether someone is praying for them or not. As a result, the standards of rigorous randomized clinical trials can be applied to study the effects of intercessory prayers on patient outcome.

Intercessory Prayers and Clinical Outcome

Medical literature is full of conflicting reports regarding the effects of intercessory prayers on clinical outcome. Some studies report that intercessory prayer has a positive outcome while other studies report no statistically significant effect. In this section, both representative positive and negative outcome studies are discussed.

Intercessory Prayers with Positive Outcome

Byrd is the first investigator who scientifically studied the effect of intercessory prayers in coronary care unit patients. He designed a prospective, randomized, double-blind protocol and randomly assigned 393 patients admitted to the coronary care unit over a ten month period to either an intercessory prayer group (192 patients) or to a control group (201 patients). While hospitalized, the first group of patients received intercessory prayers from participating Christians praying outside the hospital while patients in the control group did not receive any prayer. At the beginning of the study, there was no significant difference between the two groups of patients regarding clinical conditions, and after entry, all patients received standard medical care and follow-up care during their hospital stay. The patients in the prayer group showed significantly less complications compared to patients in the control group. The control group patients required ventilatory assistance, antibiotics, and diuretic medications more frequently than patients belonging to the intercessory prayer group. The author concluded that intercessory prayer to the Judo-Christian God has a beneficial therapeutic effect in patients admitted to the coronary care unit.[5]

Harris et al. also studied effect of intercessory prayer on clinical outcome of patients admitted to the coronary care unit. The authors randomly divided patients into either the prayer group or the control group at the time of admission. The first names of patients were given to a team of outside intercessors who prayed for these patients daily for four weeks. Patients were unaware that they were being prayed for and the intercessors never met any patients. Based on a study of 524 control group patients and 466 prayer group patients, the authors observed that the total length of patients' stay in the hospital did not differ, but patients in the prayer group had less complications based on lower MAHI-CCU (Mid-America Heart Institute-Cardiac Care Unit) scores.[6] These scores are based on the need for antianginal agents, antibiotics, or other medications (score 1 or 2), need for a temporary pacemaker or another device (score 3), need for a pacemaker or other permanent device (score 4), or cardiac arrest (score 5). The highest score of 6 indicates death. As expected, lower scores indicate fewer complications.

In another study, Leibovici randomly divided 3,393 patients with bloodstream infections either into a control group or a group to receive remote intercessory prayers. Both groups of patients were similar clinically at the time of dividing them into groups. The mortality was 28.1% in the prayer group and 30.2% in the control group. Although mortality was only slightly lower in the prayer group, the length of stay in the hospital and duration of fever was significantly lower compared to the control group. Strikingly, the maximum hospital stay was 165 days in a patient in the prayer group but 320 days in a patient in the control group. The author concluded that remote retroactive intercessory prayers were associated with a shorter hospital stay and a shorter duration of fever in patients with a bloodstream infection, and that intercessory prayers may be adopted as a complementary modality in clinical settings.[7]

Although studies cited above showed effects of remote intercessory prayers on health outcome, Matthews et al. studied the effect of in-person intercessory prayers on outcome in patients with rheumatoid arthritis using forty patients with a mean age of 62 years. All patients were taking medications for arthritis. Patients receiving six hours of in-person intercessory prayers showed significant overall improvements even in one year follow-up. The authors concluded that in-person intercessory prayers may be a useful adjunct to medical treatment for certain patients with rheumatoid arthritis.[8]

In another study, Vannemreddy et al. observed that patients with prayer habits recovered better following severe head injury.[9] Ratnasingam described a case of twenty-one-year-old man who sustained a severe head injury while rollerblading without a helmet. Based on clinical assessment, the patient was not expected to regain consciousness, but following intensive medical treatment and intercessory prayer to Saint Luigi Guanells, the patient unexpectedly recovered and his brain function during a six-month follow-up showed all normal values.[10]

Hughes described a case where the healing effect of prayer can be documented scientifically. During a routine Pap smear examination of a married woman with three children, atypical squamous cells were detected, indicating a premalignant state. She went to another clinic for a colposcopy examination (a follow-up for an abnormal Pap smear test) when a sample of cells were removed from her cervix. When she returned to the clinic to get her results, she was told that nothing abnormal was found from her examination. Interestingly, after receiving the bad news about her Pap smear, the woman talked to the pastor's wife and requested prayer. The entire congregation gathered around her to pray, hands outstretched, while the pastor touched her forehead with oil and prayed. As they prayed, the woman was overwhelmed and felt a tightening in her cervical area that she described as a gentle pulling and squeezing that was firm but not painful. She felt that was the moment of her healing. It was unlikely that her first Pap smear showed false positive results because she has a history of cervical cancer in her family. Her grandmother also developed cervical cancer; however, after prayer, her grandmother's cancer also disappeared.[11]

Intercessory prayers can improve the spiritual well-being of cancer patients. Olver and Dutney, based on a study of 999 cancer patients, concluded that intercessory prayers are effective in significantly improving overall well-being of patients with cancer, including spiritual well-being.[12] Coruh, based on a review of five randomized clinical trials investigating the effects of intercessory prayers on a patient's outcome, concluded that religious intervention, such as intercessory prayer, may improve the success rate of in vitro fertilization. Moreover, such prayers may also decrease the length of hospital stay and duration of fever in septic patients. In patients with rheumatoid arthritis, prayers may reduce anxiety and improve quality of life. Moreover, prayer may also decrease adverse outcomes in patients with cardiac diseases.[13] Five diseases where intercessory prayer may improve health outcome are summarized in Table 6.2.

Studies Showing No Effects of Intercessory Prayer

Roberts et al., based on four studies, concluded that there was no evidence that intercessory prayer had any effect on numbers of people dying from leukemia or heart diseases.[14] Benson et al. studied the effects of intercessory prayer on clinical outcomes following coronary artery bypass graft (CABG) surgery. The authors reported that complications occurred in 52% patients (315 out of 604 patients) who received intercessory prayers versus 51% (304 out of 597 patients) who did not receive any prayer. The authors concluded that intercessory prayer had no effect on recovery after CABG surgery.[15] In another published report, Roberts et al. reviewed ten studies involving 7,646 patients and concluded that intercessory prayer had no effect on the mortality of patients.[16] Walker et al. observed no benefit of intercessory prayer on treatment outcome in patients enrolled in an alcohol rehabilitation program.[17] Mathai and Bourne reported that intercessory prayers had no effect in the treatment outcome of children with psychiatric disorders.[18]

Spirituality and Better Survival in Patients with AIDS

Acquired immune deficiency syndrome (AIDS) is caused by infection with HIV (human immunodeficiency virus), most commonly spread through unprotected sex or the sharing of contaminated needles during IV drug abuse. Following initial infection, a person may experience a brief period of influenza-like illness, but few or no symptoms may be noticed for several years. This is the chronic stage of HIV infection when the HIV virus is replicating in the body. If an HIV infection is detected at this stage and treatment is initiated, survival can be prolonged for many years. However, if HIV infection is undetected or untreated after the initial infection, the HIV viral load reaches a high level after ten to twelve years and the patient then suffers from AIDS and has severely compromised immune function. Patients with AIDS are susceptible to opportunistic infections that will eventually kill them. HAART therapy (highly active antiretroviral therapy) has significantly improved survival rates of patients with AIDS. However, approximately one million people still die worldwide each year due to AIDS.[19]

Austin et al. commented that intercessory prayer or distant healing has no significant effect on clinical outcome of patients with AIDS.[20] However, spirituality has a positive effect on the survival of patients infected with HIV. Ironson and Kremer reported that spiritual transformation occurs in approximately 39% patients with HIV. Based on a study of 147 HIV infected patients, the authors observed that a spiritual transformation was associated with a better treatment outcome (undetectable viral load and higher CD4 count indicating better immune function), better adherence to medicine, fewer symptoms, less distress, positive coping, and better attitudes towards life (existential transcendence, optimism, and death acceptance). More strikingly, survival up to five years (follow-up period in the study) was 5.35 times more likely in patients with spiritual transformation compared to patients with no spiritual transformation. The authors concluded that a spiritual transformation was associated with a better clinical outcome in patients with HIV infection.[21]

In one study involving 177 patients living with HIV, the Kremer et al. observed that 65% of patients had positive spiritual coping, 7% had negative coping and 28% had no significant spiritual coping. The authors observed that positive spiritual coping was associated with a sustained, undetectable viral load and higher CD4 count over four years. The authors concluded that the association between positive spiritual coping and immune preservation was direct (not explainable by viral load suppression), suggesting potential psychoneuroimmunological pathways. The authors concluded that positive spiritual growth is an important area of intervention to achieve an undetectable viral load and reduce the progression of disease. Moreover, spiritual growth in these patients also was shown to prevent substance abuse.[22]

In another study involving 101 patients with HIV infection and four years of follow-up, Ironson et al. observed that patients with a positive view of God (as benevolent or forgiving) showed a lower viral load and higher CD4 count compared to patients with a negative view of God (as harsh, judgmental, or punishing). Patients with a negative view of God showed faster progression of disease over a period of four years. Results remained significant even after adjusting for church attendance and psychological variables. The authors concluded that belief in a loving and forgiving God is associated with a better health outcome in patients with HIV infection.[23] Positive effects of spiritual transformation on survival of patients with HIV are summarized in Table 6.3.

How Prayer Works

There are several hypotheses proposed by scientists to explain how prayers work (Table 6.4). Prayer may be viewed as a complementary and alternative therapy because prayer, along with standard medical care, may produce better results than standard medical care alone. The principle behind prayer is the belief that God or a higher being is willing to listen to our petitions, and prayers may result in God's intervention to produce desired healing that may be incomprehensible from our current knowledge of medicine.

Placebo Effect

Many scientists argue that healing power of prayer is a placebo effect. *Placebo* is a Latin word meaning "I shall please." In medical research, a placebo is used to study the effects of a medicine where a group of randomly-selected subjects receive a fake medicine (placebo) while another group of subjects receive the real medicine. Subjects do not know whether they receive the real medicine or placebo. To be considered successful, the effect of the real medicine must be significantly better than the placebo effect. A placebo effect may also be defined as positive, unexpected effect when a subject receives a fake medicine or a fake treatment.

The reason for a placebo effect is a patient's recovery expectations, because the patient does not know that he or she has received a fake medicine. In this case, a patient's body chemistry may be altered to produce the desired effect, or it may be related to capacity of the human mind to alleviate a physical condition, such as the perception of pain. Because prayer has no medicinal value, the positive effect of prayer may be due to placebo effect. However, some scientists concluded based on their research that the healing effect of prayer cannot be explained from a simple placebo effect. For example, in one study based on 219 women who were undergoing in vitro fertilization/embryo transfer, the pregnancy rate was 50% in women who received distant intercessory prayers compared to 26% in women who did not receive any prayer. Patients were blinded to whether or not they received prayers.[24] Such data is difficult to explain simply from the placebo effect.

Another hypothesis is that prayer acts as a relaxation response to patients. The relaxation response is the opposite of the stress response. Yoga, meditation, and prayer can produce a relaxation response, which counteracts adverse clinical effects of stress on disorders such as hypertension, anxiety, insomnia, and aging. The relaxation response reduces the expression of genes linked to inflammatory responses and stress-related pathways.[25]

Positive Emotion Hypotheses

Positive emotion may be responsible for health benefits of prayer. These positive emotions include feelings of peace, joy, hope, faith, trust, and love. The hypothalamic-pituitary system in the brain is responsible for linking positive thoughts with the release of messenger molecules in the blood, which in turn render positive health effects. Prayer also stimulates the human immune system and hormonal system, which may aid in healing. Lutgendorf et al., based on a study of 5,576 elderly subjects, reported that religious participation more than once a week was associated with elevated IL-6 (interleukin-6), indicating a boost in the immune system. Moreover, attending religious services was associated with significantly lower mortality in a twelve-year period.[26] Meditation and yoga have positive effects on human cardiovascular systems. Prayer may have a similar effect. Mody studied the effect of a Hindu prayer (Surya Namaskar, or sun prayer) on cardiovascular health and concluded that such prayers may significantly improve cardiac functions.

Prayer Acts as a Channel for Supernatural Intervention

Although science does not deal with God, all hypotheses presented so far fall short of explaining the healing effects of prayers. As a result, some investigators consider the healing effect of prayer a result of supernatural intervention. In general, science deals with naturalistic explanations only and supernatural intervention goes beyond the reach of science. However, undeniably, most people turn to prayer with a belief that a divine being who transcends the natural universe hears and responds to prayer. Koening described a case of an eighty-three-year-old woman that illustrates belief in supernatural intervention. The woman suffered from a rare pain condition (poly motor and sensory neuropathy) due to complications from her diabetes. She also had hypertension and goiter. Her pain was resistant to all medications, including steroid injections. The woman said that when she experienced severe pain, she prayed, which always eased her pain. Eventually, prayer was her primary source of pain relief.[28] Faith in God may be a key factor in understanding how prayers render healing effects.

Quantum Entanglement and Related Hypotheses

Quantum entanglement is an interesting hypothesis to explain how prayer may work. Quantum entanglement is a phenomenon described by Einstein as "spooky action at a distance." In quantum entanglement, two subatomic particles (for example, two electrons separated by a distance) can act in a similar fashion, as if they are connected or communicating. However, no known science can explain such a phenomenon." This is very similar to the concept of telepathy, where two individuals are separated but they can mentally communicate with each other. This phenomenon is rarely found among humans, but in the sub-atomic level, this phenomenon is not so uncommon. Knowing that sub-atomic particles are building blocks of this universe, one can loosely interpret that quantum entanglement is a phenomenon that connects everything within the universe, and so we are all connected to each other. Leder commented that the human mind is non-local in nature (not confined in the human brain only, but also in part belongs to the universe) and during distant healing, a healer can be connected to the person requiring healing through some mechanism related to quantum entanglement. A similar mechanism may explain the phenomenon of telepathy and other psi phenomena.[29]

Rading, using thirteen pairs of volunteers (eleven pairs of adult friends and two mother-daughter pairs) who were separated by twenty meters and had no apparent way of communicating, showed that in three out of thirteen pairs, when one person was stimulated, the other person in the pair also reacted because both subjects showed very similar brain waves as recorded by EEG (electroencephalogram). The authors concluded that under certain conditions, the EEG of an isolated human subject can be similar to the EEG of another person who is a part of the pair. This phenomenon suggests the presence of an unknown form of energetic communication between two subjects who are separated from each other.[30]

If an isolated pair can communicate through an unknown form of energetic communication, it is also possible to communicate with God through this unknown mechanism related to quantum entanglement. Near-death studies have shown that human consciousness may survive physical death because human consciousness is separated from the brain and exists in the universe. If a patient can be resuscitated then the consciousness can come back to the physical brain. Therefore, a non-local human consciousness may be in quantum entanglement with omnipresent God, and petitions made to God through prayer may or may not be answered based on God's decision. However, for many scientists, God is an enigma belonging to the realm of religion, not science.

Various Types of Healing

Other than physical therapy, which is a scientifically valid method for treatment for a variety of conditions, including rehabilitation after stroke or heart attack, there are many other complementary modalities of healing. Acupuncture, massage therapy, aromatherapy, Reiki and healing touch have health benefits. Many people use such modalities for improving health and emotional well-being. Reiki healing may also be adopted for distance healing. In this section, effects of touch healings and distant healings on health outcomes are discussed.

Health Benefits of Reiki

Reiki is a form of energy therapy where a therapist may lightly touch a person or work with the energy field of the person by moving hands just over the physical body. The purpose of this healing modality is to transfer energy from the universe to the recipient so that body can be in a self-healing mode. The Reiki principle is based on the principle of universal life force energy, which is available to anyone who is willing to be in tune with this source of energy. Reiki was discovered in Japan in the late nineteenth century in Japan by a Buddhist monk, "Usui." Reiki can be practiced in the first or the second level, but the highest level—or the third level of practice skill—is usually achieved by Reiki masters only. A complete Reiki session may take twenty to thirty minutes and a Reiki therapist may place his or her hand on twelve to thirteen positions on the whole body. Reiki therapy is a cost-effective, non-invasive therapy without any side effects. Such holistic therapy can be easily adopted in a variety of clinical situations and may be a valuable nursing intervention.[31]

Burnout is a common phenomenon among health care physicians working at mental health clinics. In one study, Rosade et al. the showed that Reiki intervention for thirty minutes was very effective in reducing the burnout phenomenon among community mental health clinicians.[32]

In a study by Bukowski et al. involving a nine-year-old female child with a history of stroke, seizures, and type 1 diabetes (insulin dependent diabetes), six weeks of Reiki treatment by a Reiki Master resulted in a positive change in sleep pattern (better sleep during 33.3% of nights) and no reports of seizure during Reiki treatment. The Reiki Master reported that child was relaxed within five to seven minutes of Reiki treatment. Bukowski et al. concluded that Reiki is helpful adjunct therapy for children with increased stress level and sleep disturbances.[33]

Olson et al. conducted a randomized clinical trial to study effect of Reiki on the pain management of twenty-four cancer patients and observed that patients who received pain medication along with Reiki showed significantly lower perception of pain, lower diastolic blood pressure, and decreased heart rates on days they received Reiki treatment compared to patients who received pain medication alone.[34] In a hospice patient with advanced cancer, Bullock reported relief of pain and swelling following one to two Reiki treatments per week for five months. At the time of diagnosis, his symptoms suggested that he had a very limited life expectancy, but his level of comfort and quality of life improved dramatically as a result of Reiki treatment. The author commented that Reiki has been associated with dramatic results for many patients. Some general trends seen with Reiki for patients in hospice care include periods of stabilization, in which there is time to enjoy the last days of one's life; a peaceful and calm passing if death is imminent; and relief from pain, anxiety, dyspnea and edema. The author concluded that Reiki is a valuable, complementary therapy to enhance quality of life in hospice patients.[35]

Gillespie et al. studied the efficacy of Reiki to reduce pain and improve mobility in patients with Type 2 Diabetes suffering from painful diabetic neuropathy (sever nerve pain associated with complications of diabetes). The authors observed that Reiki therapy was associated with significant pain reductions in these patients.[36] In another study, the Vitale et al. reported that women who received Reiki intervention after abdominal hysterectomy reported less pain and requested lesser amounts of pain medications compared to women who did not receive Reiki therapy.[37]

Demir et al. studied the effect of distant Reiki healing on anxiety and fatigue in cancer patients. The Reiki intervention group received thirty minutes of distant Reiki healing on five occasions. The control group patients did not receive any Reiki treatment. At the end of study period, patients in the Reiki group experienced significantly less pain, fatigue, and anxiety compared to patients in the control group. The authors concluded that Reiki may decrease pain, anxiety, and fatigue in cancer patients.[38] In contrast, Joyce and Herbison, based on systematic review of three studies, found no effect of Reiki in reducing depression and anxiety.[39]

Health Benefits of Healing Touch

Healing touch is a complementary, noninvasive biofield energy therapy that supports the body's natural healing process and enhances the immune system. Trained practitioners use their hands to manipulate energy through light touch or putting hands over certain parts of the body to balance, clear, or boost the human energy system. Healing touch therapy, like other bio-energy therapies, is rooted in concepts of compassion, positive intention, self-empowerment, and the mind-body-spirit triad. Wong et al., based on participants three to eighteen years old with cancer, showed that healing touch therapy was associated with a significant reduction in pain, fatigue, and stress in both children and their caregivers. In addition, parents' perception that their children were having pain also decreased significantly in the healing touch group compared to the control group, in which children participated in reading or play activities. The authors concluded that healing touch therapy is an effective intervention modality in pediatric oncology patients.[40]

Decker et al., based on a study of twenty older adults experiencing pain, observed that healing touch is a feasible complementary therapy for the elderly with pain.[41]

Lincoln et al. reported that both healing touch and healing harp (a form of music therapy) are effective in reducing pain, anxiety, and nausea in patients after surgery.[42]

In another study involving people with osteoarthritis, the Lu et al. observed that healing touch sessions three times per week for six weeks were associated with significant improvements in nine out of twelve outcome variables (including intensity of pain and interference of pain with activities), but people in the control group who received no healing touch but had friendly visits did not show any improvement. The reduction in joint pain and improvement in joint function in people who received healing touch therapy lasted for three weeks after the cessation of healing touch therapy. These results indicate that healing touch therapy is effective as an adjunct to medical care in people suffering from osteoarthritis.[43]

Wetzel described a case report of a woman who had a significant wound infection after cesarean birth. Following healing touch therapy, her wounds were healed faster than expected from medication alone.[44] In another study using seventy-three women, the authors observed that healing touch was effective in reducing anxiety from diagnostic breast cancer procedures.[45] Anderson et al. studied the effect of healing touch therapy on pain, nausea, and anxiety following bariatric surgery and reported that healing touch therapy significantly decreased pain, nausea and anxiety immediately after surgery and during three days post-surgery in patients who received healing touch therapy compared to patients who did not receive such therapy.[46]

Umbreit reviewed applications of healing touch in acute care settings and commented that nurses are beginning to use healing touch to reduce pain and anxiety in their patients. Moreover, healing touch therapy also promotes relaxation, accelerates wound healing, diminishes depression and increases overall well-being of patients.[47]

Does Distant Healing Work?

Distant healing is a complementary and alternative medicine where a healer can induce healing in a person who is physically separated from the healer. Reiki healing can also be performed from a distance. Although difficult to explain from our current knowledge of science, there are a few scientific studies reporting positive effects of distant healing, although other studies observe no beneficial effect of distant healing. Schlitz et al. observed that subjects who had undergone reconstructive breast surgery only received positive effects of distant healing (a significantly better mood) but patients who had undergone purely elective cosmetic surgery did not receive any benefits of distant healing.[48]

Sicher et al. studied the effects of distant healing on forty patients with AIDS. Patients were matched for age, CD4 count, and AIDS related symptoms and then randomly selected either to receive ten weeks of distant healing or receive no healing. Healers and patients never met. After six months, the authors observed that patients who received distant healing had fewer AIDS-related symptoms, lower disease severity, fewer visits to physicians, fewer hospital admissions, and fewer days of hospitalization (if hospitalized) compared to patients in the control group. Patients who received distant healing also scored higher on the positive mood scale (twenty six versus fourteen in the control group), but no difference was found in CD4 count between these two groups.[48]

Astin et al. reviewed a total of twenty-three clinical studies involving 2,774 patients to investigate efficacy of distant healing and reported that thirteen studies (57%) reported a positive outcome of distant healing, while nine studies showed no such effect and one study showed negative effects of distant healing.[49] Walach et al., using 409 patients with chronic fatigue syndrome, studied the effectiveness of distant healing and reported that distant healing had no mental or physical benefit to these patients.[50]

How Complementary Healing Modalities May Work

For touch based healing, sympathetic arousal during a healing touch may be responsible for the feeling of well-being. The slight stimulation of the skin by the slow, stroking movement of the healer's hand may also trigger nonspecific treatment effects by enhancing bond and trust between the healer and the subject receiving such treatment. Pleasant touch can also cause emotional response as a result of release of hormone oxytocin, especially in female subjects. A Reiki session can result in changes in systolic blood pressure, electromyography (a diagnostic technique recording electrical activities of skeletal muscles), and skin temperature indicative of relaxation. Based on a study using twenty-two subjects, the authors observed that relaxation and well-being increased significantly after a healing touch session. The authors concluded that higher sympathetic arousal during a touch-based healing is associated with an overall feeling of improved well-being in a subject after such treatment.[51]

The mechanism of distant healing is not clear. Distant healing has some similarity with prayer because many distant healers are also religious or spiritual and often pray before a session. As a result, hypotheses related to how prayer works may also be applicable to explain how distant healing works, from the placebo hypothesis to quantum entanglement.

Conclusion

Many studies have shown a positive health outcome of prayer, although some studies found no effect of prayer on patient outcome. However, prayer is a non-invasive, safe, complementary alternative medicine with no side effects. As a result, depending on the religious and spiritual beliefs of a patient, individual or intercessory prayers may be recommended as an adjunct healing modality. Reiki and healing touch also have healing effects, especially in improving overall well-being of patients. There are some studies showing positive effect of distant healing on patients. These complementary and alternative approaches are non-invasive and free from any side effects.

Table 6.1 Five categories of health related prayers

Category of prayer	Comments
Disease-centered prayer	This type of prayer is directly related to the patient's illness and is the most common type of prayer. Prayers may be intended for healing or for gaining mental strength to cope with illness.
Assurance-centered prayer	This is the second most common type of prayer and provides confidence to patients that God will take care of them during illness despite their wrongdoings in life. Prayer for protection prior to surgery also falls under this category of prayer.
God-centered prayer	God-centered prayer is focused on relationship between God and the patient. This type of prayer is a prayer of adoration where recovery from an illness may be a secondary issue.
Other-centered prayer	In this type of prayer, a patient prays for others, such as family members, so that they have strength and faith during the patient's illness. Prayer may also be for the physician who is treating the patient.
Lamentations	This is the least common type of prayer, where a patient may experience fear or doubt for recovery.

Table 6.2 Top five diseases where intercessory prayer may significantly improve health outcome

Clinical Condition/Disease	Comments
Patients with cardiovascular diseases admitted to coronary care unit	Control group patients required ventilatory assistance, antibiotics, and diuretic medications more frequently than patients who received intercessory prayers
Patients with bloodstream infections, including sepsis	Reduced mortality and length of stay in the hospital
Cancer patients	Improved spiritual wellbeing and a case report of the disappearance of cervical cancer
Patients with head injury	Better recovery and a case report of unexpected complete recovery
Patients with rheumatoid arthritis	Improvement in clinical condition

Table 6.3 Positive effect of spiritual transformation on survival of patients with HIV

- Lower or undetectable viral load
- Higher CD4 count indicating better immune function
- Survival up to five years may be 5.35 times more likely among patients with spiritual transformation compared to patients with no spiritual transformation.
- Better compliance with medications
- Fewer symptoms
- Less distress and positive life attitude
- Belief in a benevolent and forgiving God is associated with a better outcome compared to believing in a punishing or judgmental God

Table 6.4 Proposed hypotheses to explain how prayer works

- Placebo effect
- Relaxation response of prayer
- Prayer as an expression of positive emotion
- Prayer activating the immune system and hormonal system, causing healing
- Prayer may have a positive effect on cardiovascular system
- Prayer as a channel for supernatural intervention
- Quantum entanglement

Chapter 7
Yoga, Meditation, Religiosity and Spirituality are Associated with Happiness

Introduction

Happiness is a positive emotional state of mind which is related to life satisfaction. In scientific terms, happiness is often referred as "subjective well-being." In 1984, Dr. Diener defined three ways to look at subjective well-being:

- Life satisfaction
- Positive affect (positive emotion)
- Negative affect (negative emotion)

Positive affect is a subjective mental state of pleasurable engagement with environment, while negative affect includes worries, sad feelings, and anxiety. A person who scores high on the subjective well-being scale has high life satisfaction and frequently experiences positive emotions. Diener et al. commented that in general, a happy person feels negative emotions, including worries, infrequently. A happy person is more productive in his or her job, interacts positively with other members of the society, and in general has a healthier life than an unhappy person. Genetic makeup, personality type, cultural variables, social support, resources, and life circumstances all affect subjective well-being.[1] Personality factors such as extroversion, positive self-esteem, optimism, the ability to bond with others, and an internal locus of control all contribute to happiness. Scientists have developed objective ways of studying subjective well-being using different questionnaires with values assigned to each question for assessment. This way, a numerical score can be generated to study subjective well-being in a group of individuals. The Oxford Happiness questionnaire, Subjective Happiness Scale, Satisfaction with Life Scale, Panas Scale, Subjective Well-being Inventory Score, and Subjective Well-Being survey created by the Organization of Economic Cooperation and Development are used by many investigators to objectively measure subjective well-being of participants in various studies.

The happiness of a person can also be assessed by measuring biochemical parameters, such as levels of salivary cortisol, fibrinogen stress response, blood pressure, heart rate, and possibly immune function. Less stress in life is correlated with happiness and subjective well-being. Salivary cortisol, blood pressure, and heart rate are increased in response to stress. Moreover, brain activity also correlates with positive or negative affect. Layard concluded that while positive affect is correlated with activity of the left dorsolateral prefrontal cortex, the negative effect is correlated with activity of the right dorsolateral prefrontal cortex.[2]

Does Money Increase Happiness?

Although the GDP (gross domestic product) is widely held to be correlated with citizens' welfare, Richard Easterlin reported that Americans did not become happier during 1946–1970, a period of rapid economic growth in the United States, and this phenomenon is known as "Easterlin's paradox." This paradox indicates that citizens of the wealthiest countries are not always happiest.[3] According to World Happiness Report 2013, the happiest country was Switzerland. Canada ranked 5th and Mexico ranked 14th, ahead of U.S., which was 15th place. Moreover, in last fifty years, the happiness of Americans did not change, but in European countries, the level of happiness increased with increased economic growth. Work is necessary to pay bills, and good earnings contribute to a person's self-esteem, but the number of hours an average American works per week exceeds average number of hours a European works per week. Because Americans spend more time at work, it cuts into time spent connecting with friends, family, and romantic partners. Research has indicated that people are most happy during socialization and during an intimate relationship with a romantic partner, while people are least happy during commuting to work and during working hours. Therefore, working long hours to make more money does not translate into more happiness, but spending time with loved ones or spending time to make social connections is strongly associated with greater happiness.[4]

Income appears to have a surprisingly modest impact on an individuals' happiness. According to the "experience-stretching hypothesis," mundane joys of life such as sunny days, cold beer, and chocolate bars may have greater impact on happiness than dining in a very expensive restaurant. Quoidbach et al. reported that money impairs people's ability to savor positive emotions and experiences of daily life. The authors observed that wealthier individuals reported lower savoring ability (ability to enhance and prolong positive emotional experience). Moreover, the negative impact of wealth on an individual's ability to savor undermines the positive impact of money on the person's happiness.[5] Dunn et al. reported that people who spend money on others are happier than people who spend money for themselves.[6]

Although money does not buy happiness, poverty is not desirable because it may negatively impact life. Recent research already starts to distinguish two aspects of subjective well-being. The emotional well-being, or experienced happiness, refers to the emotional quality of a person's everyday experience and everything that makes it pleasant or unpleasant, including the frequency and intensity of experiencing joy, fascination, and affection as well as anxiety, sadness, or anger. Life evaluation is another aspect of subjective well-being where a person is asked how satisfied he/she is with the life overall. Based on a survey of more than 450,000 people, Kahneman and Deaton reported that although emotional well-being increases with income at lower levels, beyond an annual income of $75,000, there is no significant change in emotional well-being with increasing income. The authors commented that although low income exacerbates the emotional pain associated with divorce, ill health, and being alone, further increases in income above the $75,000 threshold no longer improve overall emotional well-being. However, the authors also mentioned that their finding does not mean that if an individual's salary increases from $100,000 to $150,000 the person will be unhappy. The authors concluded that high income buys life satisfaction but not happiness.[7]

Effective Approaches for Stress Relief

Stress is a part of everyday life but it also negatively affects the physical and emotional well-being of a person. Although yoga, meditation, church attendance, and spiritual growth are associated with stress release, increased emotional well-being, and happiness, there are also other effective ways of stress release. In this section, these alternative approaches for stress release are discussed briefly.

Men and women react differently in response to stress. In general, women have better coping skills than men in terms of dealing with stress. In contrast to men, who prefer the "fight or flight" approach to stress, women prefer the "tend and befriend" approach in response to stress.[8] Tending involves nurturant activities designed to protect the woman and her offspring from stress, while befriending is the creation and maintenance of a social network that may provide a safety net. Studies have indicated that the hormone oxytocin which is secreted from the brain in conjunction with female reproductive hormones may be related to different patterns of responses of women to stress. During stress, cortisol and epinephrine increase the blood pressure, but oxytocin can counteract the action of cortisol.

Interaction with family members and friends is a good way to reduce stress.[9] According to the buffer hypothesis, social support or a social network may improve mental health by buffering the negative effect of stress. Olstad et al. studied this hypothesis and concluded that total social support or a social network buffered the deteriorating effect of the total stressor score on the mental health of subjects. The effect was stronger in women than men. Interestingly, social support or social networks also have a significant buffer effect against work-related stress.[10]

Laughter and a good sense of humor are associated with stress reduction and good health. Laughter provides a physical release for accumulated tension. Laughter can effectively reduce stress and also has a positive effect on the immune system.[11] Pet ownership has many health benefits, including a significant reduction in stress levels. A pet acts as a "social catalyst" and facilitates interpersonal interactions. Wells studied the behavior of 1,800 strangers towards a female experimenter and observed that when the experimenter was alone, strangers ignored her, but when she was in the company of a dog, she got the most attention from these strangers.[12] Cortisol is a stress hormone, and blood concentration of cortisol usually increases in response to stress. Human-animal interaction can reduce the cortisol level in plasma. In one study, the authors observed a reduction in plasma cortisol in subjects after they petted their own dog or even an unfamiliar dog, but when they read quietly, there was no reduction of plasma cortisol.[13] Cat ownership also has beneficial effects on stress reduction and the reduction of blood pressure.

Being physically active reduces the risk of all-cause mortality. Woodcock et al. commented that thirty minutes of daily, moderate intensity activity for five days a week (two and a half hours per week) was associated with a 19% reduction of all-cause mortality compared to no physical activity. In addition, seven hours per week of moderate activity reduced all-cause mortality by 24%.[14] In 1995, the American College of Sports Medicine and Centers for Disease Control and Prevention published a national guideline for physical activity, and later, the American Heart Association endorsed that guideline. The primary guideline is that all healthy adults between the ages of eighteen and sixty-five need moderate-intensity physical activity for a minimum of thirty minutes each day, five days a week or vigorous intensity physical exercise for at least twenty minutes a day, three days a week. The combination of moderate and vigorous intensity activity is also acceptable. Physical activity as well vigorous exercise increases heart rate and is beneficial for health.[15]

Aromatherapy can significantly reduce stress. In one study, twenty-two healthy volunteers who sniffed lavender or rosemary oil for five minutes showed higher free radical scavenging capacity and lower cortisol level in saliva, indicating that aromatherapy can reduce stress and improve the antioxidant defense of the human body. Interestingly, lavender can increase the antioxidant capacity of saliva in much lower concentrations than rosemary.[16]

Massage also has a direct relationship with health outcome because a patient's perception of stress and anxiety are significantly reduced after massage. The simple act of touch-focused care and even a five minute hand and foot massage can be useful in lowering a patient's perceived level of stress.[17]

Music is also effective in lowering stress. Cervellin and Lippi commented that experimental evidences now suggest that some kind of music might modulate different cardiac and neurological functions, thus reducing stress. This effect is also known as the Mozart effect and may be useful as a therapeutic tool for reducing stress in both healthy individuals and ill subjects.[18]

Making love to a spouse or partner is a great way to reduce stress levels. A study by Burleson et al. based on 58 middle-aged women (mean age 47.6 years) who recorded physical affection, different sexual behavior, stressful events, and mood ratings every morning for 36 weeks found that physical affection or sex with a partner on a day correlated with a higher positive mood the following morning, indicating that physical intimacy is effective in reducing stress.[19] Men can also get stress release from sex. However, sexual misadventure increases risk of sexually transmitted diseases, including the possibility of getting infected with HIV virus.

Leisurely activities and taking vacations can reduce stress at least on a short term basis. Grump and Matthews performed a large study with 12,338 subjects on the effect of vacations on all-cause mortality in middle-aged men with a high risk of cardiovascular disease for a study period of nine years. They concluded that the frequency of annual vacations by these middle-aged men was associated with a reduced risk of all-cause mortality and, more specifically, mortality associated with cardiovascular diseases.

The authors concluded that vacationing is good for the health.[20] Various effective ways of stress release are listed in Table 7.1.

Yoga and Happiness

In Chapter 4, the effects of yoga on stress release is discussed in detail, while in Chapter 5, the effectiveness of meditation in reducing stress is discussed. Moreover, the practice of yoga enhances muscular strength and body flexibility, promotes and improves respiratory and cardiovascular function, improves sleep patterns, and reduces stress, anxiety, depression, and chronic pain, all of which are correlated with subjective well-being and an improved quality of life.[21] Yoga is not simply an exercise protocol. Yoga integrates both body and mind, thus enhancing spiritual growth. Because spiritual growth is also associated with increased emotional well-being and happiness, it is expected that people who practice yoga on a regular basis are also happier in life.

Well-being in the workplace is characterized by employees who perceive themselves to be happy and experience positive emotional states, such as joy, pleasure, and being productive. Resilience to stress indicates that employees can respond productively when faced with significant changes or pressure to achieve an outcome. In a study based on forty-eight employees in a British University, Hartfiel et al. showed that six weeks of yoga intervention consisting of one sixty-minute class per week was associated with marked improvements of feeling joy, energy, and confidence compared to subjects who were placed on the waitlist. The authors concluded that yoga is an effective tool for achieving resilience to stress among employees in a stressful workplace. Moreover, yoga also improves emotional well-being and elation among employees.[22] Sharma et al., based on a study of seventy-seven subjects who practiced yoga for only ten days, observed that yoga was associated with remarkable improvement in feelings of happiness and interpersonal relationships, as evidenced by higher scores on the "subjective well-being inventory score" (SUBI) in the participants of yoga group only. There was no statistically significant change in SUBI scores among people who did not participate in yoga.[23] Malathi et al. also reported higher SUBI score in subjects who practiced yoga compared to subjects in the control group. The authors concluded that yoga practice can make a person happier and improve overall subjective well-being.[24]

Overall psychological well-being consists of both hedonic and eudaemonic happiness. Hedonic happiness reflects subjective well-being, which consists of satisfaction in life, general well-being, expectation-achievement congruence, transcendence, family support, and social support for an individual. Eudaemonic aspects of well-being consist of purpose of life, growth, and understanding of the meaning of life. Based on a study of 124 subjects, Ivtzan and Papantoniou observed that practice of yoga increased both hedonic and eudaemonic happiness. Moreover, the number of years of practicing yoga was also associated with higher gratitude and meaning of life scores.[25] Bussing et al., based on a study of 160 subjects, observed that intensive yoga practice increased practitioners' spirituality, mindfulness, and positive mood.[26]

Reed studied the positive effect of a single Hatha yoga session using forty-five subjects who participated in yoga and twenty-five subjects who attended a lecture (control group). All subjects completed the revised Morningness-Eveningness Questionnaire (rMEQ) prior to the yoga session or attending lecture. The rMEQ consists of questions about usual wake time, time of peak energy, and tiredness. Usually, scores range from 4 to 25 with scores of 4-11 indicating an evening person, 12-17 indicating the person is neither a morning nor evening person, and scores 18-25 indicates that the person is a morning person. In addition, all subjects participated in the Visual-Analog Mood Scale (VAMS) to record scores before and after yoga intervention (or attending lecture). The VAMS is a measure of positive mood of an individual. A person is asked to make a vertical tick mark on a 100-millimeter horizontal line with the anchors "very, very sad" on the left, "neutral" in the center and "very, very happy" on the right. The score is in the range of 0 (left anchor) to 100 (right anchor) and the actual score depends on the distance of the tick mark in millimeter from the left anchor. The authors observed that in the yoga group, 33% of subjects were the evening type, 25% were the morning type, and 42% were neither type. In the control group, 24% of subjects were the evening type, 36% were the morning type, and 40% were neither type. Interestingly, in the control group, VAMS did not change at all after attending the lecture (mean pre-score: 41.00, post mean score: 41.54). In sharp contrast, VAMS scores were significantly higher after yoga class (mean pre score: 55.59, post mean score 69.68), indicating that yoga is associated with a better positive mood and increased happiness. Moreover, greater changes in VAMS scores were observed after yoga in evening persons. The authors concluded that Hatha yoga is effective in improving the positive mood of a person.[27]

Yoga is associated with increased level of GABA (gamma-aminobutyric acid), a neurotransmitter in the brain. Streeter et al. studied brain GABA level using magnetic resonance spectroscopic imaging in eight yoga practitioners and eleven control subjects. The authors reported a 27% increase in GABA levels in yoga practitioners after a sixty-minute yoga session, but no change was observed in the subjects in the control group who participated in the sixty-minute reading session.[28] GABA is an inhibitory neurotransmitter that slows down the firing of neurons and creates a sense of calmness. Moreover, low levels of GABA are associated with depression and anxiety. Therefore, increased GABA levels may explain why participants experience tranquility and happiness after a yoga session. Moreover, increased GABA levels after yoga also explain why yoga is effective in alleviating symptoms of anxiety and or depression. Interestingly, drugs that are used to treat anxiety and depression also increase brain GABA level.

Yoga is effective in reducing serum cortisol level. Cortisol is a stress hormone and reduced levels of cortisol after yoga indicate that yoga is effective in reducing stress (see Chapter 4). In a study based on seven yoga instructors, Kamel et al. observed that fifty minutes of practice of yoga was associated with mean reduction of serum cortisol level from a pre-yoga value of 11.69 microgram/dL to post yoga value of 9.75 microgram/dL. Interestingly, alpha brain waves were also increased after yoga sessions.[29] Alpha brain waves are associated with a relaxed state of mind. Individuals are also creative during alpha brain wave activity. Froeliger et al. reported less reactivity to negative images in the right dorsolateral prefrontal cortex in yoga practitioners compared to subjects in the control group.[30] Higher activity of right dorsolateral prefrontal cortex is associated with negative feelings. Factors that may be associated with increased subjective well-being in yoga practitioners are summarized in Table 7.2.

Meditation and Happiness

Like yoga, meditation has many positive effects on health and also improves the emotional well-being of a person. The Oxford Happiness Questionnaire was developed by psychologists Peter Hills and Michael Argyle at Oxford University.[31] This questionnaire is widely used by scientists to measure the subjective well-being of a person. The questions in the Oxford Happiness Questionnaire are listed in Table 7.3 along with information about interpreting the score. In one study, Ramesh et al. investigated effect of Raja Yoga meditation on positive thinking, which is an index of self-satisfaction and happiness in life. The authors used the Oxford Happiness Questionnaire and observed that in a group of twenty-five meditators, the average score was 4.66 (a score over 4 indicates that a subject is happy), but the average score among twenty-five non-meditators was 3.98. There were no significant differences in age, marital status, education, employment status, or economic status between individuals in both groups. More interestingly, only one individual in the meditation group out of 25 subjects was unhappy while eleven subjects in the non-meditator group were unhappy. The authors commented that such differences were statistically significant and concluded that the Raja Yoga meditation practice significantly increased self-satisfaction and happiness in life.[32]

Mind-wandering, a common activity during awake state, is associated with lower levels of happiness in life. Therefore, lowering mind-wandering may increase happiness in life. Mind-wandering is associated with the brain function known as "default mode network." This network is also associated with attention lapses, anxiety, attention deficit hyperactivity disorder and other clinical disorders. Therefore, changing this default mode of the brain activity may increase happiness in life. Interestingly, experienced meditators report less mind-wandering compared to non-meditators. Brewer et al. commented that the main nodes of default-mode networks in the brain are relatively deactivated in experienced meditators across all meditation types. Therefore, a meditator experiences joy and happiness in life.[33]

Meditation has positive effects on brain function and plasticity (see Chapter 5). EEG (electroencephalograph) studies have shown asymmetric patterns in subjects after meditation, indicating positive emotion in meditators compared to subjects in the control group. Tang et al., using forty undergraduate students, observed that short-term meditation (one thirty-minute session each day for five days) induced higher positive mood and lower negative mood states than relaxation training alone. A brain imaging study showed no difference in cerebral blood flow before the study, but after the study, subjects who meditated showed enhanced blood flow in the left anterior cingulate cortex, and such activation of left prefrontal cortex region of the brain is related to positive emotion.[34] Dopamine is a neurotransmitter which is also called the "reward molecule" of the brain. Kjaer et al., using PET imaging of the brain, observed that meditation increases dopamine levels in the brain.[35]

Religiosity, Spirituality and Happiness

Based on a study of 500 undergraduate students, Tkach and Lyubomirsky observed that one of the predictors in these students was religion.[36] Various predictors of happiness are listed in Table 7.4. Diener et al. estimated that approximately 68% population on the earth (4.6 billion people) would say that religion is important in their daily lives. Moreover, studies have found that in general, religious people have a higher subjective well-being. The association of religiosity with a higher subjective well-being is mediated by social support and increased understanding of the meaning of life. However, there is a paradox: if religion makes people happy, why are people in developed countries dropping out from religious practice? The authors commented that in nations with more difficult life conditions, people are more religious because in these nations, religiosity is associated with greater social support, respect, and understanding of the meaning of life.[37] Using Gallup World Poll data, Oishi and Diener observed that although life satisfaction was substantially higher among people living in wealthy nations than poor nations, the understanding of meaning of life was higher among people living in poor countries because people in these nations are more religious.[38]

Green and Elliott reported that individuals who identify as religious tend to report better health and happiness regardless of religious affiliation, religious activities, work, family, social support, and financial status.[39] Berthold and Ruch studied 20,538 participants and observed that people with religious affiliation who also practiced their religion were more satisfied with their life and scored higher on the meaning of life scale than non-religious people or people who passively belonged to a religious group. Moreover, people who practiced their religion showed several character strengths, including more kindness, love, gratitude, hope, forgiveness, and spirituality. Interestingly, the authors found no difference between people belonging to a religious group who did not practice their religion and people without any religious affiliation. The authors concluded that individuals only get benefit from belonging to a religious affiliation if they participate in religious practice.[40]

Maselko et al., based on statistical analyses of responses from 1,445 subjects, observed that 32% women participated in public religious activity at least once a week versus 23% men who participated at least weekly public religious activity.[41] However, both men and women engaging in public religious activities (such as attending service at a church, synagogue, or temple) at least once a week reported greater happiness and lower psychological distress. Moreover, men benefitted more from attending religious services than women. In contrast, association between private religious practices (praying or reading a Holy Text) and subjective well-being was less significant than the association between attending public religious services and subjective well-being. The authors concluded that when public religious activities, private religious activities, and spirituality were considered, public religious activities emerged as the most consistent predictor of health and wellness being among men. For women, only private religious activities were associated with higher level of happiness.

Spirituality is broadly defined as any blissful experience or positive emotion in a person who focuses on people but not on himself or herself. Spirituality is associated with a greater purpose of life and may or may not include believing in God. Although most religious people are also spiritual, a spiritual person may not be religious. However in certain religions—for example, in Buddhism—the concept of "God" does not exist in original teachings. Because religion is associated with happiness and most religious people are also spiritual, it is obvious that spirituality is associated with happiness and greater meaning of life. Vaillant considered positive emotions such as awe, love and attachment, trust and faith, compassion, gratitude, forgiveness, joy, and hope to be associated with spirituality, and further argued that spirituality is also associated with activities of the limbic system of the brain.[42]

Research has indicated a positive association between spirituality and emotional well-being. Spirituality is positively associated with gratitude, forgiveness, and empathy. Both religiosity and spirituality can protect an individual from depression and alcohol or substance abuse. In a large study involving 3,966 adolescents and young adults as well as 2,014 older adults, Barton et al. observed that there was a positive correlation between spirituality and positive emotion among 83% of the adolescents and young adults studied. Moreover, such association was also observed among 71% of the older adults. The level of depression was also negatively correlated with spirituality in both groups of subjects. Moreover, spirituality also protected these subjects from substance abuse.[43]

Conclusion

Both yoga and meditation are associated with better physical and emotional health. Moreover, both practices can increase spirituality. As a result, people who practice yoga and meditation are, in general, happier in life. Religion has many beneficial effects in human life and in general, people who participate in religious activities are happier regardless of denomination, but passive association with a religion is not associated with increased happiness in life. Neurobiologically, the human brain is wired to be spiritual, and as expected, spirituality is associated with positive emotions and increased life satisfaction.

Table 7.1 Various approaches to reduce stress by developing healthy habits

- Social networking/interacting with friends and family members
- Good sense of humor
- Pet ownership
- Exercise/physical activities
- Yoga and meditation
- Volunteering/community activity
- Religion/spiritual growth
- Six to eight hours of good night sleep
- Aromatherapy and massage
- Music therapy
- Sex with spouse/partner
- Leisurely activity and vacation

Table 7.2 Factors that may be associated with increased subjective well-being in yoga practitioners

- Better health due many positive health effect of yoga (see Chapter 4)
- Increased antioxidant effects contributing to positive health (see Chapter 4)
- Reduced levels of stress and anxiety
- Lower serum cortisol
- Higher brain GABA levels
- Higher activity of alpha brain waves
- Less reactivity in the right dorsolateral prefrontal cortex

Table 7.3 Oxford happiness questionnaire, scoring method and interpretation of result

Oxford Happiness Questionnaire*
I don't feel particularly pleased with the way I am (-)
I am intensely interested in other people (+)
I feel that life is very rewarding (+)
I have very warm feelings towards almost everyone (+)
I rarely wake up feeling rested (-)
I am not particularly optimistic about the future (-)
I find most things amusing (+)
I am always committed and involved (+)
Life is good (+)
I do not think that world is a good place (-)
I laugh a lot (+)
I am well satisfied with everything in my life (+)
I don't think I look attractive (-)
There is a gap between what I would like to do and what I have done (-)
I am very happy (+)
I find beauty in some things (+)
I always have as cheerful effect on others (+)
I can fit in everything I want to (+)
I feel that I am not especially in control of my life (-)
I feel able to take anything on (+)
I feel fully mentally alert (+)
I often experience joy and elation (+)
I do not find it easy to make decisions (-)
I do not have a particular sense of meaning and purpose in my life (-)
I feel I have a great deal of energy (+)
I usually have a good influence on events (+)
I do not have fun with other people (-)
I don't feel particularly healthy (-)
I do not have particularly happy memories of the past (-)

*[31] Hills P, Argyle M. The Oxford questionnaire: a compact scale for the measurement of psychological well-being. Personality Individual Differences 2002; 33: 1073-1082.

	Scoring method	Total score/ Interpretation
	Question related to positive emotion (+) should be scored as: Strongly disagree (score 1) Moderately disagree (score 2) Slightly disagree (score 3) Slightly agree (score 4) Moderately agree (score 5) Strongly agree (score 6) Questions related to negative emotion (-) should be scored as Strongly agree (score 1) Moderately agree (score 2) Slightly agree (score 3) Slightly disagree (score 4) Moderately disagree (score 5) Strongly disagree (score 6)	Total score is obtained by adding the individual scores for questions 1–29 and dividing that score by 29 **Interpretation:** Lowest score 1 (very un-happy) to highest score 6 (very happy). In general, a score over 4 indicates an overall happy state of the person.

Table 7.4 Eight unique predictors of happiness

Strongest Predictors	Comments
Direct attempts	Direct attempts to happiness are proactive behaviors such as smiling and acting happy. Expressions of emotion also heighten happiness.
Social affiliation	Social activities are associated with happiness.
Religion	Praying and performing religious rituals are associated with emotional well-being. Religious activities also increase social connectedness and meaning of life. Religious practice may protect an individual from drug or alcohol abuse.
Partying	Partying increases social connection, but extroverted people gain more from partying and club activities than introverted people.
Active leisure	Exercise or engagement in a hobby contributes positively to happiness.
Other Predictors	
Goal pursuit	Striving to accomplish certain things or reach a career goal is associated with increased subjective well-being.
Passive leisure	Passive leisure activities such as watching TV or playing a video game or card game contribute to happiness.
Mental control	Mental control such as not expressing one's emotions or negative thoughts are negatively associated with happiness.

Bonus Section

Scientific Investigations on Medical Miracles

Introduction

The modern scientific method originated with three English intellectuals: Bacon, Locke and Newton. Under their influence, physicians at the University of Edinburg in late eighteenth century articulated the view that medicine is a secular profession with no appeal to divinity. Scientific explanations are materialistic, and according to science, God must always remain an enigma. From the scientific point of view, cosmos (the universe) is unemotional, mechanistic, directionless, and uncaring as it continues to repeat cause and effects following natural laws. Therefore, science believes that all natural phenomena can be explained by these laws, leaving no place for a miracle.[1] The word miracle comes from the Latin word *miraculum* meaning amazing or astonishing. According to the Oxford Dictionary of World Religions, a miracle is defined as a "striking event brought about, usually by God, for religious purpose, against the usual course of nature." A miracle is a gift of loving God who breaks natural laws to perform a miracle and then restores such laws. Therefore, miracles should be hoped for, but not expected by a faithful believer.

Medical Wonders Versus Medical Miracles

It is important to differentiate medical wonders from medical miracles. Medical wonders are fruits of talented scientists' medical research and have been occurring for centuries, starting from Edward Jenner's 1798 discovery of the small pox vaccination following his observations that milkmaids who previously came into contact with cowpox had immunity against small pox.

Later, Lois Pasteur discovered the principles of vaccination, microbial fermentation, and pasteurization. He also created the first vaccines for anthrax and rabies. In 1923, Banting and Macleod were awarded the Nobel Prize in Physiology or Medicine for the discovery of insulin. The discovery of insulin revolutionized the treatment of diabetes, especially type 1 diabetes, where patients had previously been destined to die. Penicillin was initially discovered by Alexander Fleming and later developed by Howard Florey and Ernst Chain. It's known as a miracle drug and was the first antibiotic available for treating microbial infections. There are many wonders of medical science including the discovery of anesthesia and analgesia, identifying germs causing infection, present knowledge of immunity, knowledge of preventing sepsis, understanding human physiology with knowledge of symptoms, organotherapy (for example treating diabetes with insulin), and discovery of vitamins.[2] More recently, organ transplantation, artificial hearts, prosthetic organs, and advanced techniques of life support are also examples of medical wonders. Important medical wonders are listed in Table 8.1.

Breakthroughs in emergency medicine have enabled science to halt and even reverse death. When heart stops, a person stops breathing and his or her brain wave (EEG) becomes flat. At that moment, a person is pronounced dead, but it may take several hours for cells inside the body to die, and that is the reason death could be reversed by wonders of modern medicine in some patients. A three-year-old girl who had fallen in an icy pond and was not discovered for thirty minutes was finally brought to a hospital and was put on an ECMO (extracorporeal membrane oxygenation) machine capable of maintaining artificial circulation and kidney function. The girl miraculously survived despite being pulseless and apneic with no oxygen or circulation for a long period of time. Although such miracles could be attributed to technological wonders of medical science, such advancements have inadvertently led science into a domain that was traditionally viewed as the domain of theology and religion.[3] Many patients who had clinical deaths reversed by physicians have described their amazing near-death experiences.

In this chapter, medical miracles are discussed. There is no straightforward definition of a medical miracle, but in general, it is assumed that it is a medical miracle when a very sick patient or a patient with an incurable disease recovers from illness without any plausible medical explanation. However, accepting a medical miracle may be a difficult challenge to a physician because the realm of miracles is left out from medical school curriculums and medicine is primarily driven by scientific materialism. Professor Victor S. Sierpina, MD, the Laura Nell Nicholson, Family Professor of Integrative Medicine at the University of Texas Medical Branch at Galveston, commented, "Although the realm of supernatural including miracle is routinely left out from modern medicine, yet every doctor in practice for any significant amount of time has experienced the occurrence of mystery and unexplainable in the lives of his or her patients. There are cases of spontaneous healing which could not be explained by knowledge of contemporary medicals science."[4]

Dr. Sierpina described his experience with an eighty-one-year-old woman who had a bad fall. Based on her swelling and lack of mobility, Dr. Sierpina was convinced that she had broken her humerus (the long bone running from the shoulder to the elbow) and he ordered an X-ray. While she was waiting for her X-ray, Dr. Sierpina's staff was arranging for the woman to see an orthopedic surgeon to fix her broken arm. When the X-ray report was available, Dr. Sierpina was amazed to find out that there was no fracture. When he told the good news to her patient, she told Dr. Sierpina that she was praying fervently on her way to the radiology department and her prayer had the desired effect.

In another case report, Steve, a ten-year-old boy suffering from bone cancer in his leg, refused to undergo amputation to save his life (it was the only treatment available, according to the oncology experts). Many years later, a researcher on spontaneous healing found Steve alive and cancer free. Dr. Sierpina commented, "While I certainly do not recommend ignoring a doctor's advice, especially with a life threatening disease like cancer, in this case, something miraculous happened. No one, not even the patient and the family had the least idea how his unexpected survival might have transpired. Maybe miracles are normal, natural, and occur all the time, and only our failure to believe in them keeps us from recognizing how regularly they occur."[4]

Near-Death Experiences

What happens when people die has intrigued human beings throughout time. However, with the wonders of modern medicine, death can be reversed and near-death recollections have been reported by millions of patients. The first comprehensive, modern report about near-death experiences was published in 1975 by Raymond Moody, PhD, MD, in his international best seller, "Life after Life."[5] This book contains 150 cases of near-death experiences, and Dr. Moody identifies fifteen characteristics of near-death experiences described by survivors who had close encounters with death. Dr. Moody defined near-death experience as "any conscious, perceptual experience occurring in individuals pronounced clinically dead or who came close to death."

Common features of near-death experiences include an overwhelming feeling of joy and peace, no pain, an out of body sensation, passing through a tunnel and then coming in contact with bright light, communication with dead relatives, life review, and finally back to the physical body. One of the most compelling pieces of evidence that near-death experiences may be glimpses of heaven is the positive transformation of many individuals who had near-death experiences. Most individuals become more spiritual or religious and do not have a fear of death. In his later book, "Life Beyond," published in 1989, Dr. Moody extensively studies nearly 1,000 case reports of near-death experiences when people nearing death experienced going through a tunnel and then coming to bright light and meeting angelic beings of light, feeling eternal joy and peace which they had never experienced before in their life.[6] Anyone can have a near-death experience, including young children and people blind from birth.

Near-death experiences are profoundly mystical, spiritual, or religious in nature, and such experiences have long-term positive transformational effects in the lives of individuals who have such experiences. Many people who have had a near-death experience report less fear of death, a greater sense of altruism and empathy, selflessness, less materialism, increased faith, a deeper understanding of the meaning of life, and becoming more spiritual. In one published report, the author studied thirty-seven patients for six months who had out-of-hospital cardiac arrest. Out of thirty-seven patients, seven patients (18.9%) had near-death experiences. The author observed that patients who had near-death experiences had higher tolerance for others, a greater concern with social justice, higher senses regarding inner meanings of life, and a greater appreciation of nature compared to patients who did not have near-death experiences.[7]

There are many scientific theories that attempt to explain near-death experiences from known scientific knowledge of neurobiology. These theories include:

- Anoxia of the brain (absence of oxygen supply to the brain)
- Involvement of temporal lobe
- Drug-induced near-death experience
- Endogenous endorphins (morphine-like compounds produced by the human brain) or neuro-transmitter serotonin
- Centripetal ischemia of the retina (reduced or lack of oxygen supply to the retina)
- Other neurobiological mechanism
- Psychological interpretations

However, none of these theories can explain near-death experiences reported by blind people. Moreover, children around three years old are not primed with the concept of the afterlife, but near-death experiences of young children are similar to adult near-death experiences. In addition, people with near-death experiences transform positively, have no fear of death, and some of them gain amazing psychic gifts. In contrast, people facing life-threatening experiences with no near-death experiences do not overcome fear of death or transform spiritually. Therefore, near-death experiences may be considered a unique miraculous experience where a person may get a glimpse of heaven.

My Mother's Recovery: I Witnessed a Medical Miracle

My mother had a life threatening illness in June 2011 with multiple organ failure. After my cousin informed me that my mother was on life support with less than a 1% chance of recovery, I took the next available flight and arrived at Calcutta (now Kolkata, India) on June 18. After talking to the attending physician we decided to continue the life support for two more days so that my wife, Alice, could get a chance to say goodbye to my mother. Alice arrived at Kolkata a little after midnight on June 20 and we had special permission to see my mother at the hospital. When we arrived, the resident physician informed me that the medical team reviewed my mother's case and if we agreed, her life support would be discontinued next morning. Alice was in tears and she started to pray from her Christian prayer book. After a half hour, my mother opened her eyes for the first time in one week. Her pain reflex came back and the resident physician was perplexed. We decided to continue her life support as there was some hope. The next morning, the attending physician was totally surprised to see my mother's progress in last eight hours. After another two weeks of hospitalization, my mother recovered fully and she is still alive. The attending physician and his colleagues considered my mother's complete recovery to be a miracle. My mother later told us that she saw my wife with two beautiful women dressed in white robes standing by her side, but Alice had come to Kolkata alone.

Investigating Medical Miracles

After my mother's miraculous recovery, I started searching for reports of medical miracles using PubMed, a large database of medical literature maintained by the NIH (National Institute of Health). This is the largest database of medical literature used by most medical professionals for education and research. When I searched the database using the phrase "medical miracle," 272 articles were found. Out of these, I critically studied twenty-five articles because they appeared to deal directly with reports of medical miracles. Some of these papers discussed research reviewing canonization files of the Vatican's Secret Archives, which I address in the later part of this section. The other 247 papers provided some explanation for unexpected recoveries or discussed miracle drugs or medical procedures that authors considered to be wonders of medical science. However, knowing many medical professionals do not like the phrase "medical miracle," I also searched for "unexpected complete remission of cancer" and found eighty-seven articles. On closer review, I identified fourteen papers where patients had complete remission of cancer that was totally unexpected based on their prognosis.

Musella et al. reported an unexpected complete remission of advanced vulvar adenocarcinoma (cancer of the vulva) in a woman after treating her with the common chemotherapeutic medicines platinum and paclitaxel.[8] Feng et al. reported the unexpected remission of hepatocellular carcinoma (liver cancer) with lung metastasis, a bad prognosis, in two patients treated with thalidomide and cyproheptadine (drugs used to stop skin itching).[9] Nuzzo et al. reported a case of a young man who was suffering from liver cancer and resected brain metastasis with an expected survival of six to nine months. He had a complete remission for six years following chemotherapy with dacarbazine, cisplatin and vinblastine (all common anticancer drugs).[10]

Miracles and the Vatican

The pope proclaims a saint with the word *discernimus,* which translates to "we recognize it," but canonization is a long process which occurs after beatification, for which at least one miracle is required (only God can work miracles, but the saint can intercede on the behalf of those who appeal to him or her). For canonization, at least two miracles are required, although martyr saints are exempt from such a requirement. The records of miracles are carefully constructed to serve the canonical tradition and such documents are a part of the Vatican's secret archive, a privileged source of social, religious, cultural, and medical history. Historical records demonstrate that in the canonization process from 1200 to 1500 AD, medical men actively appeared as witnesses, and in the second half of the thirteenth century, many canonization processes included at least one medical man who witnessed or provided expert testimony to rule out the possibility that there was a medical explanation for a miraculous cure. Physicians also play a crucial role in the modern canonization process, as a panel of five distinguished physicians living in Rome meet every fortnight between mid-October and mid-July to examine miracles and render their judgment on whether the cure was natural or inexplicable by known scientific knowledge. A decision by the majority of the panel that the cure was scientifically inexplicable could be considered a miracle, but the pope has the final authority to determine if such an event was a miracle.[11]

Professor Jacalyn Duffin, MD, a highly reputed hematologist, was asked to review a set of bone marrow aspirations without any clinical information about the patient. Dr. Duffin concluded based on these slides that the patient was suffering from a severe form of leukemia and must be dead. She thought that she was reviewing these slides in the context of a lawsuit. Later, she found out that the patient was still alive, and although the patient received aggressive chemotherapy in a university hospital, she attributed her miraculous cure to the intercession of Marie-Marguerite d'Youville, a Montreal woman had died two hundred years ago. This case became the capstone in d'Youville's canonization and she was the first saint born in Canada.[12]

Later, Dr. Duffin had the privilege to examine more than six hundred miracle records in the canonization files of the Vatican's Secret Archives from the seventeenth century to the twentieth century from a medical standpoint. The vast majority of these miracles were healings from physical illness (medical miracles) and nearly all accounts of miracles included testimony of one or more physicians. Only 4.4% of miracles were non-medical. Medical miracles include recoveries from cancer, orthopedic problems, neurological issues, and other illness, including tuberculosis. At the time there was no treatment for tuberculosis and death was inevitable. A miraculous cure from a mental illness was rarely documented. In the nineteenth century, avoiding surgery recommended by a surgeon but still being cured was a common form of miracle. Duffin concluded from her research that medicine, doctors, and science are key points to the Vatican's process of investigating miracles. For the Vatican, miracles occur when the patient recovers from certain death or permanent disability following excellent medical care, though physicians claim that medicine had nothing to do with the cure. Duffin further stated that many of the miracles occurred in people who had already received their last rites. A religious miracle defies explanation by science and traditionally arrogant medicine must confess its ignorance.[13]

The first miracle of late Pope John Paul II was attributed to healing of a French nun sister Marie Simon-Pierre from Parkinson's disease in 2011. Her recovery after praying to the late pope's intercession had no medical explanation because Parkinson's disease is incurable. The Telegraph, a newspaper published in the U.K., reported on June 19, 2013, that late Pope John Paul II was recognized for his second miracle when a Costa Rican woman was cured from a severe brain injury after her family began praying to the memory of the late Polish pope. Doctors testified that her healing could not be explained from scientific principles. Approval of the second miracle of Pope John Paul II indicates that he may catapult into sainthood faster than anyone else in recent history.[13]

On October 19, 2003, Pope John Paul II beatified Mother Teresa of Calcutta, who died in 1997, because the pope recognized the healing of an Indian woman as a miracle. It involved a non-Christian woman in India who had a large abdominal tumor which disappeared one day when she woke up following prayers to Mother Teresa from the Missionaries of Charity (founded by Mother Teresa). Mother Teresa may also achieve sainthood if a second miracle can be recognized by the Vatican where a fifty-six-year-old Salesian priest based in Guwahati, India, was inexplicably healed of a painful ureter stone the day before his scheduled surgery. The surgeon was surprised to discover the disappearance of the stone when a pre-surgery X-ray was taken. There was no evidence that the patient passed the stone in his urine and the surgeon concluded that the disappearance of the stone was a miracle.[14]

Miracles of Lourdes

Between February 11 and July 16, 1858, Marie Bernarde Soubirous, an uneducated fourteen-year-old girl born in a very poor family in Lourdes, France, had eighteen visions of the Virgin Mary at Massabielle Grotto. Later, she took vows to become a nun and died in 1879. She was canonized in 1933. Thirteen cases of cures were reported in 1858 and the local bishop regarded seven of these cures as miracles. Since then, millions of people have traveled there with hopes of a miraculous cure. In 2008, the 150th anniversary of the vision of Virgin Mary, approximately nine million people visited Lourdes. Sixty-seven cures that occurred in Lourdes have been acknowledged by the Roman-Catholic Church as miracles. Moreover, in 1954, an International Medical Committee comprised of twenty skilled specialists and university professors of medicine reviewed many documents and certified twenty-six events as miraculous cures. Francois et al. examined twenty-five such cures acknowledged between 1947 and 1976 and concluded that the Lourdes phenomenon, extraordinary in many respects, still awaits scientific explanation. The Lourdes phenomenon concerns both science and religion.[15]

Medical Miracles Reported in Medical Journals

Medical miracles are also reported in mainstream medical literature when the recovery of a patient cannot be explained from current knowledge of medicine. Joyce Martin, RN, NP, a family nurse practitioner, reported a medical miracle on a New Year's Day. A boy who had been accidentally shot by his brother with a 0.22-caliber rifle was brought to the hospital.[16] The nurse tried to place an endotracheal tube (a tube placed through mouth to restore respiration), but his vocal cord was not visible due to blood in his airways. His pulse was thirty beats per minute, indicating he was collapsing and could die anytime unless put on life support. The nurse prayed according to her Christian belief and surprisingly, the tube could be placed easily during her fourth attempt. Finally, the patient's pulse and blood pressure were normalized.

The trauma surgeon operated on the boy, and after becoming stable, he was transferred to a regional hospital. However, his odds of survival were still poor, and even if he survived, he would certainly be impaired. The next day, the boy had taken a turn for the worse. Joyce Martin prayed for the patient, and two days later when she went to see him, the excited staff reported that the boy was improving and he perked up between eleven and twelve o'clock on Sunday during church hours. Nine days after the accident, the boy recovered and asked for a hamburger. The boy had three near-death experiences, and during the last experience, he was told by his grandfather to go back because it was not his time. The medical team believed the survival of the boy was a miracle.[16]

Nath et al. published a scientific paper entitled, "Miracle still happens: a rare case of self-inflicted penetrating injury of ear" where the authors describe a patient who had a sharp nail transverse the entire thickness of the skull and the pointed end of the nail could be traced at opposite temporal area of the brain. Removing the nail posed a great danger, as it was already impacted inside the skull bone, and if the patient survived, there would be hearing impairment and substantial brain damage. Miraculously, the patient recovered after surgery without hearing loss or brain damage, which could not be explained by current principles of medical science.[17] Dr. Susan Gold of Pennsylvania State University Hershey Medical Center reported the miraculous survival of a patient who had heart failure due to infarction (heart attack). The patient also suffered from kidney and liver failure along with sepsis. The patient was placed on an ECMO (Extracorporeal Membrane Oxygenation) machine but later recovered fully. The author concluded that the patient's survival was a miracle.[18]

Jane T. Broxterman, MD, a faculty member of the University of Kansas School of Medicine reported the miraculous recovery of a seventy-three-year-old man who was found unconscious in his driveway. His CT scan showed a large subdural hematoma (blood clot in the brain). His condition deteriorated six hours later, but the family declined emergency craniotomy because despite successful surgery, his quality of life would be poor. The family requested the medical team to provide comfort care to the patient. The palliative care team was consulted and he was started on propofol and fentanyl (a narcotic analgesic) for comfort. However, twelve hours later the nurse reported to Dr. Broxterman that the patient was able to squeeze her hand, which was totally unexpected from a dying patient. Dr. Broxterman asked the nurse to discontinue infusion of both medicines and when the effects of these medicines faded, the patient responded to the doctor's verbal commands and his physical condition improved dramatically, which was not consistent with his CT scan result. One hour later, the patient was able to sit on a chair and the neurosurgeon arrived to order another CT scan. When the neurosurgeon read the CT scan, he was astonished to discover that the subdural hematoma was almost resolved. Over the next several days, the patient continued to improve, and, after spending a total of eighteen days in the hospital and rehabilitation center, the patient recovered completely. At the time of the report, he was still living at home, driving, enjoying life, and learning to play guitar. The author acknowledged that recovery of the patient was a miracle and that the experience changed her as a physician and as a person.[19]

Dr. Kirkpatrick reported the miraculous recovery of a patient who suffered from cardiac arrest and, later, a seizure. Dr. Kirkpatrick informed the patient's wife that he may have sustained severe hypoxic brain damage (brain damage due to inadequate supply of oxygen) during his cardiac arrest, but the wife told the physician that she expected the complete recovery of her husband because of the power of prayer. To the utter surprise of Dr. Kirkpatrick, the patient recovered completely and the patient's wife said that she spent all night at a prayer vigil and was convinced that the recovery would be complete. Dr. Kirkpatrick commented that since then, he has witnessed several recoveries in the intensive care unit which could also be described as miraculous.[20]

However, a miracle may not only be an unexplainable cure from a life threatening illness, but also the peaceful acceptance of death as integral part of life; overcoming the fear of death is also a miracle. Michael, an eighteen-year-old boy who was suffering from metastatic osteosarcoma (cancer that originated in a bone but spread to other organs) had undergone a limb-salvage procedure, but the primary tumor responded very poorly to chemotherapy. In the following months, his cancer had spread to other organs, including his brain, despite aggressive chemotherapy, and the physician was running out of options. However, Michael was still upbeat and hoping for a miracle, although his parents agreed with the physician and accepted palliative care instead of a potentially fruitless aggressive medical intervention, such as putting him on a ventilator. However, Michael wanted to live and requested the doctor do anything to keep him alive and Michael's girlfriend had the same request. Michael's condition continued to deteriorate with the development of respiratory failure, but later that night, Michael was peaceful and did not want to go to ICU. He passed away peacefully that night. Morales La Madrid, his physician commented that Michael's eventual acceptance of his impending death was a miracle, because without that miracle, his suffering would be unnecessarily prolonged.[21]

Spirituality, Religion, and Medical Practice

Spirituality and religion are related, but may differ conceptually. A spiritual person conducts his or her life in relation to the question of transcendence, while a religious person believes in a religious book, rituals, and practices that a particular religion recommends for connecting with God. Spirituality and religion have an impact on a patient's ability to cope with illness. In a paper published in Medical Journal of Australia, Jantos and Kiat considered prayer as a medicine (see Chapter 6).[22]

Unfortunately, the interrelationship between spirituality and medical sciences has been viewed with suspicion for centuries. In fact, spirituality and religion are often regarded as foreign elements in current medical practice. Ghadirian commented that during the last two decades, there has been an upsurge of interest in the role of spirituality in medical practice in North American universities because many patients with life-threatening or chronic diseases expect their health care professionals to address or at least acknowledge their spiritual concerns.[23] Although "spirituality" or "religion" may not be included as a check box on a physical examination note, physicians should be more involved with patients, discussing spirituality or religious beliefs to foster a better physician-patient relationship.[24]

Miracles and Palliative Care

Marie Bernadette Soubiroud (1844-1879), a Christian mystic and saint, commented, "Our God sends miracles only extremely rarely." Miracles should not be considered a regular event in life. However, when breaking bad news to a patient or family many physicians hear, "Thanks Doctor, but I am hoping for a miracle and fully expect that it will happen." For many dying patients, God's healing energy and divine intervention are the ultimate treatment option when all medical care fails to produce any recovery. In one survey, 57% of respondents believed that God's intervention could save a family member even if a physician had declared that treatment would be futile. Even one in five health care professionals in the survey believed that God could reverse a hopeless outcome. This is a big dilemma for physicians, especially those dealing with patients in the cancer ward, neonatal ICU, critical care ICU, and emergency room who must decide when to withdraw life support as a family is waiting and praying for a miracle. Savulescu and Clarke argued that in the case of a terminally-ill patient receiving life support with a family hoping for a miracle to happen, the continuation of life support could be justified if the patient's family is willing to pay for such expensive treatment. However, when family members request to use a publicly funded medical facility to wait for a miracle, then physicians and hospital administrators are faced with a difficult dilemma.[25]

Howard DeLisser, MD, of the University of Pennsylvania School of Medicine published a paper discussing a practical approach to the family waiting for a miracle. This approach involves exploring the meaning and significance of a miracle with family members, providing a balanced, non-argumentative response and negotiating patient-centered compromise while still respecting spiritual and or religious beliefs of family members. Such an approach tailored to each specific family can be effective in helping a family accept the inevitable death of their loved one. However, when there is a continued insistence on therapy because a miracle is expected, the physician should enter into further discussion with family members to identify a mutually-accepted middle path between the demands of the family members for full medical care and the recommendation of the physician which involves comfort care. Ideally a compromise should be reached where the family members do not feel marginalized but the physician still has the sense of providing meaningful medical care. In case such compromise cannot be reached, the ethics committee of the hospital or a conflict resolution expert of the institution should be involved.[26] Dr. DeLisser suggested several approaches a physician may take to discuss care of a patient with family members expecting for a miracle. These approaches are summarized in Table 8.2.

Cooper et al. commented that few medical professionals have formal training in responding to family members who say they are hoping for a miracle." The authors suggested that physicians should do their best to preserve the hope, dignity, and faith of family members while presenting medical issues in a helpful and non-confrontational way. The authors presented an acronym, AMEN, as a useful tool to negotiate patient care with patient or family members:

- A for affirm: Affirm the position with patient/family that the physician is hopeful too.
- M for meet: Meet with the family members and saying something like, "I join you in hoping (or praying) for a miracle."
- E for educate: However a physician must educate family members discussing medical issues of the patient from a scientific view point.

- N for no matter what: Assure the patient and family members that no matter what, the physician will stay with them in every step of care.[27]

Brierley et al. reviewed 203 cases over a period of three years involving end-of-life decisions. In 186 out of 203 cases in which withdrawal or limitation of invasive therapy was recommended by medical teams, the outcome was accepted by family members. However, in the remaining seventeen cases, extended discussion with medical teams and local support mechanisms did not lead to resolution. Of these cases, eleven involved explicit religious claims that intensive care should not be stopped due to expectation of divine intervention and complete cure. The distribution of religions of family members included Protestants, Roman Catholics, Muslims and Jews. Five of these eleven cases were resolved after meeting with respective religious community leaders. One child had intensive care withdrawn following a court order, but for the remaining five cases, no resolution was possible due to expressed expectations that a miracle would happen.[28]

Carlos E. Pavia, PhD, MD, an oncologist, commented that in dealing with a family hoping for miracle for a dying patient, he would say, "Since God is an all-powerful being, He can perform a miracle anywhere and at any time. Whether you're in the ICU or the ward, being treated with chemotherapy or whether the cancer remains untreated." The authors agreed that in patients with advanced cancer under palliative care, the expectation of a miracle is often a difficult point for health professionals in the process of restructuring care and preparing for end-of-life comfort measures. The authors recommended that it is better not to enter into a religious dispute with family members, but to make an interdisciplinary approach involving psychiatrists and other professionals to resolve issues of end-of-life care. The authors also commented that grief could be less painful for those family members who have faith.[29]

Conclusion

Although medical miracles do not happen every day, I was surprised to hear that several of my friends and colleagues who are experienced physicians and deal with critically ill patients every day have witnessed at least one or two accounts of miraculous recoveries which could not be explained scientifically. However, miracles do not occur every day, as all humans are mortal. For family members hoping for miracle, the best approach is to respect the medical opinion of the physician, talk to a religious leader of the community, and pray for a miracle, but at the same time, accept the reality.

Table 8.1 Examples of medical wonders

- Discovery of small pox vaccine
- Discovery of microorganisms and pasteurization process
- Discovery of X-ray and radiology
- Discovery of insulin to treat diabetes
- Discovery of penicillin
- Discovery of various antibiotics, including drugs such as aminoglycosides and vancomycin to treat life threatening illness
- Discovery of oral contraceptives
- Discovery of antivirals including antiretroviral agents to treat AIDS
- Remarkable advances in treating patients with cancer
- Modern advances in anesthesia techniques and pain management
- Advances in surgery and organ transplantation
- Modern advances in imaging techniques (MRI, PET scan)
- Tracheal intubation and advanced airway management techniques to support life
- Pacemaker and artificial heart
- Kidney dialysis
- Survival of infants with a very low birth weight
- Prosthetic devices
- Genetic testing and personalized medicine

Table 8.2 A practical approach by a physician to a family expecting a miracle

Approach	Comment
Emphasize non-abandonment	The care team should be attentive to the patient even in the setting of conflict or disagreement with the family regarding patient care. In case of conflict, physicians may unconsciously withdraw and or distance themselves from either the patient or the family, sending a message of abandonment. This must be avoided.
Cite professional obligation	When death is near, there is no professional requirement that the physician will base a treatment plan on the expectation of a miracle. Rather, when death is inevitable based on current medical knowledge, a physician must respectfully review his or her professional obligations with family members and the priority should be making the patient comfortable.
Reframe the meaning and manifestation of the miracle	The physician may offer the thought that miracle has already happened as bitterly estranged family members are brought together due to a patient's illness. Moreover, when a patient accepts death gracefully, surprising positive changes may be inspired in family members.
Suggest that if a miracle is going to happen, a physician's action will not prevent it	Convince the family that if it is truly in God's will that a miraculous healing will occur, then such miracle must occur regardless of action of the physician. A pastor or a clergy may be a better position to have such a discussion with the patient's family.

References

Chapter 1

1. Koening, H. G. "Research on religion, spirituality and mental health: a review." *The Canadian Journal of Psychiatry* 54 (May 2009): 283-291.
2. Smart, Ninian and Frederick Denny, ed. *Atlas of the World's Religions*. New York: Oxford University Press, 2007.
3. Schmitt, A. K., M. Danisik, E. Aydar, E. Sen, I. Ulusoy, and O. M. Lovera. "Identifying the volcanic eruption depicted in a Neolithic painting at Çatalhöyük, Central Anatolia, Turkey." *PLoS One* (January 2014): e84711.
4. Timmons, S. M. "A Christian faith based recovery theory: understanding God as sponsor." *Journal of Religion and Health* 51 (December 2012): 1152-1164.
5. Sayadmansour, Alireza. "Neurotheology: the relationship between brain and religion." *Iranian Journal of Neurology* 13 (2014): 52-55.
6. Dakubo, J. C. B., S. B. Naaeder, and R. Kumodji. "Totemism and the transmission of human pentastomiasis." *Ghana Medical Journal* 42 (December 2008): 165-168.
7. Wallace, E. R. 4th. "Freud and religion." *The American Journal of Psychiatry* 136 (February 1979): 237-238.
8. Beker, Earnest. *Denial of Death*. Free Press: 1997
9. Cicirelli, V. G. "Fear of death in older adults: prediction from terror management theory." *The Journals of Gerontology,* Psychological Sciences and Social Sciences 57 (July 2002): 358-366.
10. Henrie, J., and J. H. Patrick. "Religiousness, religion and death anxiety." *International Journal of Aging and Human Development* 78 (2014): 203-227.

11. Krause, N., and R. D. Hayward. "Religious involvement and death anxiety." *Omega* 69 (2014): 59-78.

12. Hui, V. K., and P. G. Coleman. "Do reincarnation beliefs protect older adults Chinese Buddhists against personal death anxiety?" Death Studies 36 (Nov-Dec 2012): 949-958.

13. Kunin, Seth D. *Religion: The Modern Theories*. Maryland: John Hopkins University Press, 2003.

14. McCullough, M. E., C. K. Enders, S. L. Brion, and A. R. Jain. "The varieties of religious development in adulthood: a longitudinal investigation of religion and rational choice." *Journal of Personality and Social* Psychology 89 (July 2005): 78-89.

15. Stark, Rodney and Williams Sims Bainbridge. *A theory of Religion*. New Brusnwick, NJ: Rutgers University Press, 1996.

16. Stark, Rodney. *Sociology*. 10th ed. Cenage Learning, 2006.

17. Shariff, A. F. and A. Norenzayan. "God is watching you: priming God concepts increases prosocial behavior in an anonymous economic game." *Psychological Science* 18 (September 2007): 803-809.

18. Roberts, G. "When punishment pays." *PLoS One* 8 (2013): e57378.

19. Sosis, Richard. "The adaptive value of religious rituals." *American Scientist* 92 (March-April 2004): 166-172.

20. Norenzayan, A., and A. F. Shariff. "The origin and evolution of religious prosociality." *Science* 32 (2008): 58-63.

21. McKay, Ryan, Charles Efferson, Harvey Whitehouse, and Ernst Fehr. "Wrath of God: Religious Primes and Punishment." *Proceedings of the Royal Society* B Biological Sciences 278 (November 2010): 1858-1863.

22. Sir James George Frazer. *The Golden Bough: A Study in Magic and Religion*. Simon and Brown, 2013.

Chapter 2

1. Eliade, Mircea. *Yoga: Immortality and Freedom*. Translated by Willard R. Trask. Princeton: Princeton University Press, 1969.
2. Jayaraman, V. "The origin and definition of the name Hindu." http://www.hinduwebsite.com/hinduism/h_meaning.asp. Accessed October 15, 2015.
3. Gambhirananada, Swami. *Taittiriya Upanishad*. Calcutta, India: Advaita Asrama, 2006.
4. Telles, S. and N. Singh. "Science of the mind: ancient yoga texts and modern studies." *The Psychiatric Clinics of North America* 36 (March 2013): 93-108.
5. Satchidananda, Sri Swami. *The Yoga Sutra of Patanjali*. Integral Yoga Publications: 2012.
6. Hayes, M and S. Chase. "Prescribing yoga." *Primary Care Clinic Office Practices* 37 (March 2010): 31-47.
7. Vivekananda, Swami. *The Complete Works of Swami Vivekananda*. Calcutta, India: Advaita Asrama, 1965.
8. Telles, S. and N. Singh. "Science of the mind: ancient yoga texts and modern studies." *The Psychiatric Clinics of North America* 36 (March 2013): 93-108.
9. Muktibodhananda, Swami. *Hatha Yoga Pradipika* 3rd ed. Bihar School of Yoga, 2013.

Chapter 3

1. Cook, Christopher C. H. "Religious psychopathology: the prevalence of religious content of delusion and hallucinations in mental disorders." *The International Journal of Social Psychiatry* 61 (June 2015): 404-425
2. Crick, F. and C. Koch. "Are we aware of neural activity in primary visual cortex?" *Nature* 375 (May 1995): 121-123.
3. Azari, Nina P., John Missimer, and Rudiger J. Seitz. "Religious experience and emotion: Evidence for

distinctive cognitive neural patterns." *International Journal for the Psychology of Religion* 15 (2005):263–281.

4. Carmody, Denise Lardner and John Tully Carmody. *Mysticism: Holiness East and West.* New York: Oxford University Press, 1996.
5. Waller, Niels G., Brian A. Kojectin, Thomas J. Bouchard Jr., David T Lykken, and Auke Tellegen. "Genetic and environmental influence on religious interests, attitude and values: a study of twins reared apart and together." *Psychological Science* 1 (March 1990): 138-142.
6. Sun, T. and C. A. Walsh. "Molecular approaches to brain asymmetry and handedness." *Nature Reviews Neuroscience* 7 (August 2006): 655-662.
7. Oardey, J., S. Roberts, and L. Tarassenko. "A review of parametric modelling technique for EEG analysis." *Medical Engineering and Physics* 18 (January 1996): 2-11.
8. Hofman, Michel A. "Evolution of the human brain: when bigger is better." *Frontiers in Neuroanatomy* 8 (March 2014): 15.
9. Gallagher, A. "Stature, body mass and brain size: a two million year odyssey." *Economics and Human Biology* 10 (December 2013): 551-652.
10. Felther, Garth J. O., Jeffry A. Simpson, Lorne Campbell, and Nickola C. Overall. "Pair bonding, romantic love and evolution: the curious case of *Homo Sapiens*." Perspective on Psychological Science 10 (Janurary 2015): 20-36.
11. Dunbar, R. I. "The social brain hypothesis and its implications for social evolution." *Annals of Human Biology* 36 (Sep-Oct 2009): 562-572.
12. Rossano, M. J. "The essential role of ritual in the transmission and reinforcement of social norms." *Psychological Bulletin* 138 (May 2012): 529-549.
13. Mattson, M. P. "Superior pattern processing is the essence of the evolved human brain." *Frontiers in Neuroscience* 8 (August 2014): 265.

14. Fumagalli, M. and A. Priori. "Functional and clinical neuroanatomy of morality." *Brain: a Journal of Neurology* 135 (July 2012): 2006-2021.

15. Wain, O. and M. Spinella. "Executive functions in morality, religion and paranormal beliefs." *The International Journal of Neuroscience* 117 (January 2007): 135-148.

16. Sambhava, Padma ed. and Karma Lingpa ed. *The Tibetan Book of the Dead: The Great Book of Natural Liberation Through Understanding in the Between.* Translated by Robert Thurman. Bantam Books, 1993

17. Joseph, R. "The limbic system and the soul". *Zygon: The Journal of Religion and Science* 36 (March 2001): 105-136.

18. Saver, J. L. and J. Robin. "The neural substrates of religious experience." *The Journal of Neuropsychiatry and Clinical Neurosciences* 9 (Summer 1997): 498-510.

19. Newberg, A., A. Alavi, M. Baime, M. Pourdehnad, J. Santanna, and E. d'Aquili. "The measurement of regional cerebral flow during the complex cognitive task of meditation: a preliminary SPECT study." *Psychiatry Research* 106 (April 2001): 113-122.

20. Schjoedt, Uffe, Hans Stodkilde-Jorgensen, Armin W. Geertz, and Andreas Roepstorff. "Highly religious participants recruit area of social cognition in personal prayer." *Social Cognitive and Affective Neuroscience* 4 (June 2009): 199-207.

21. Asp, E. K. Ramchandran, and D. Tranel. "Authoritarianism, religious fundamentalism and human prefrontal cortex." *Neuropsychology* 26 (July 2012): 414-421.

22. Tiger, Lionel and Michael McGuire. *God's brain.* Prometheus Books, 2010.

23. Joseph, P. G. "Serotonergic and tryptaminergic overstimulation on refeeding implicated 'enlightenment' experience." *Medical Hypotheses* 79 (November 2012): 598-601.

24. Borg, J., B. Andree, H. Soderstrom, and L. Farde. "The serotonin system and spiritual experiences." *The American Journal of Psychiatry* 160 (November 2003): 1965-1969.

25. Previc, F. H. "The role of the extrapersonal brain system in religious activity." *Consciousness and Cognition* 15 (September 2006): 500-539.

26. Sasaki, J. Y., H. S. Kim, T. Mojaverian, L. D. Kelley, I. Y. Park, and S. Janusonis. "Religion priming differently increases prosocial behavior among variants of dopamine D4 receptor gene." *Social Cognitive and Affective Neuroscience* 8 (February 2013): 209-215.

27. Hamer, Dean H. *The God Gene: How Faith is Hardwired into Our Genes*. Anchor, 2005.

28. Nilsson, K. W., M. Damberg, J. Ohrvik, J. Leppert, L. Lindstrom, H. Anckarsater, and L. Oreland. "Genes encoding for AP-2 beta and the serotonin transporter are associated with the personality character spiritual acceptance." *Neuroscience Letters* 441 (January 2007): 233-237.

Chapter 4

1. Birdee, G. S., S. T. Legedza, R. B. Saper, S. M. Bertisch, D. M. Eisenberg, and R. S. Phillips. "Characteristics of yoga users: Results of a National survey." *Journal of General Internal Medicine* 23 (October 2008): 1653-1658.

2. Hayes, M and S. Chase. "Prescribing yoga." *Primary Care Clinic Office Practices* 37 (March 2010): 31-47.

3. Dunn, K. D. "A review of the literature examining the physiological processes underlying the therapeutic benefits of Hatha yoga." *Advances in Mind-Body Medicine* 23 (Fall 2008): 8-10.

4. Saraswati, Swami Niranjanananda. *Prana and Pranayama*. Bihar School of Yoga, 2010.

5. Williams, Paul T. and Paul D. Thompson. "Walking versus running for hypertension, cholesterol and diabetes

mellitus risk reduction." *Arteriosclerosis, Thrombosis, and Vascular Biology* 33 (May 2013): 1085-1091.

6. Streeter, C. C., T. H. Whitfield, L. Owen, S. K. Karri, et al. "Effects of yoga versus walking on mood, anxiety, and brain GABA levels: a randomized controlled MRS study." *Journal of Alternative and Complementary Medicine* 16 (November 2010): 1145-1152.

7. Lin, S. L., C. Y. Huang, S. P. Shiu, and S. H. Yeh. "Effects of yoga on stress, stress adaption, and heart rate variability among mental health professionals—A randomized controlled trail." *Worldviews on Evidence-Based Nursing* 12 (August 2015): 236-245.

8. Michalsen, A., P. Grossman, A. Acil, J. Lanhorst, R. Ludtke, T. Esch, G. B. Stefano, and G. J. Dobos. "Rapid stress reduction and anxiolysis among distressed women as a consequence of three-month intensive yoga program." *Medical Science Monitor: International Medical Journal of Experimental and Clinical Research* 11 (December 2005): CR555-561.

9. Smith, J. A., T. Greer, T. Sheets, and S. Watson. "Is there more to yoga than exercise?" *Alternative Therapies in Health and Medicine* 17 (May 2011): 22-29.

10. Batista, J. C., A. L. Souza, H. A. Ferreira, F. Canova, and D. M. Grassi-Kassisse. "Acute and chronic effects of tantric yoga practice on distress index." *Journal of Alternative and Complementary Medicine* 21 (November 15): 681-5.

11. Woolery, A., H. Myers, B. Sternlieb, and L. Zeltzer. "A yoga intervention for young adults with elevated symptoms of depression." *Alternative Therapies in Health and Medicine* 10 (Mar-Apr 2004): 60-63.

12. Berger, D. L., E. J. Silver, and R. E. Stein. "Effects of yoga on inner-city children's well-being: a pilot study." *Alternative Therapies in Health and Medicine* 15 (Sep-Oct 2009): 36-42.

13. Huand, F. J., D. K. Chien, and U. L. Chung. "Effects of Hatha yoga on stress in middle aged women." *The Journal of Nursing Research* 21 (March 2013): 59-66.

14. Dasgupta, Amitava and Kimberly Klein. *Antioxidants in Food, Vitamins and Supplements: Prevention and Treatement of Disease.* Elsevier, 2014.

15. Yadav, R. K., R. B. Ray, B. Vempati, and R. L. Bijlani. "Effect of a comprehensive yoga based lifestyle modification program on lipid peroxidation." *Indian Journal of Physiology and Pharmacology* 49 (Jul-Sep 2005): 358-362.

16. Sinha, S., S. N. Singh, Y. P. Monga, and U. S. Ray. "Improvement of glutathione and total antioxidant status with yoga." *Journal of Alternative and Complementary Medicine* 13 (December 2007): 1085-1090.

17. Pal, R., S. N. Singh, K. Halder, O. S. Tomer, A. B. Mishra, and M. Saha. "Effects of yogic practice on metabolism and antioxidant redox status of physically active males." *Journal of Physical Activity and Health* 12 (April 2015): 579-587.

18. Tekur, P., R. Nagarathna, S. Chametcha, A. Hankey, and H. R. Nagendra. "A comprehensive yoga program improves pain, anxiety and depression in chronic low back pain patients more than exercise: an RCT." *Complementary Therapies in Medicine* 20 (2012): 107-118.

19. Cramer, H., R. Lauche, H. Haller, and G. Dobos. "A systematic review and meta-analysis of yoga for low back pain." *The Clinical Journal of Pain* 29 (May 2013): 450-460.

20. Posadzki, P., E. Ernst, R. Terry, and M. S. Lee. "Is yoga effective for pain? A systematic review of randomized clinical trials." *Complementary Therapies in Medicine* 19 (October 2011): 281-287.

21. Moonaz, S. H., C. O. Bingham 3rd, L. Wissow, and S. J. Bartlett. "Yoga in sedentary adults with arthritis: effects of a randomized controlled pragmatic trail." *The Journal of Rheumatology* 42 (July 2015): 1194-1202.

22. Sharma, M. "Yoga as an alternative and complementary approach for arthritis: a systematic review." *Journal of Evidence-Based Complementary and Alternative Medicine* 19 (January 2014): 51-58.

23. Hennard, J. "A protocol and pilot study for managing fibromyalgia with yoga and meditation." *International Journal of Yoga Therapy* (2011): 109-121.

24. Rudrud, L. "Gentle Hatha yoga and reduction of fibromyalgia related symptoms: a preliminary report." *International Journal of Yoga Therapy* (2015): 53-57.

25. Katz, J. N. and B. P. Simmons. "Carpal tunnel syndrome." *The New England Journal of Medicine* 346 (June 2002): 1807-1812.

26. Garfinkel, M. S., A. Singhal, W. A. Katz, D. A. Allan, R. Reshetar, and H. R. Schumacher Jr. "Yoga-based intervention for carpal-tunnel syndrome: a randomized trial." *Journal of American Medical Association* 280 (November 1998): 1601-1603.

27. Yusuf, S., S. Hawken, S. Ounpuu, T. Dans, et al. "Effect of potentially modifiable risk factors associated with myocardial infarction in 52 countries (the INTERHEART study): case control study." *Lancet* 364 (September 2004): 937-952.

28. Kones, R. "Primary prevention of coronary heart disease: integration of new data, evolving views, revised goals, and role of rosuvastatin in management: A comprehensive survey." *Drug Design, Development and Therapy* 5 (2011): 325-380.

29. Vijayakrishnan, R., G. Kalyatanda, I. Srinivasan, G. M. Abraham. "Compliance with the adult treatment panel III guidelines for hyperlipidemia in a resident run ambulatory clinic: a retrospective study." *Journal of Clinical Lipidology* 7 (Jan-Feb 2013): 43-47.

30. Yadav, RK, R. B. Ray, R. Vempati, and R. L. Bijlani. "Effect of a comprehensive yoga-based lifestyle modification program on lipid peroxidation." *Indian Journal of Physiology and Pharmacology* 49 (Jul-Sep 2005): 358-362.

31. Yadav, R. K., D. Magan, R. Yadav, K. Sarvottam, and R. Netam. "High density lipoprotein cholesterol increases following a short term yoga based lifestyle intervention:

a non-pharmacological modulation." *Acta Cardiologica* 69 (October 2014): 543-549.

32. Mayor, S. "Yoga reduces cardiovascular risk as much as walking or cycling, study shows." *British Medical Journal* 349 (December 2014):g7713.

33. Chu, Paula, Rinske A. Gotink, Gloria Y. Yeh, Sue J. Goldie, and M. G. Myriam Hunink. "The effectiveness of yoga in modifying risk factors for cardiovascular disease and metabolic syndrome: a systematic review and meta-analysis." *European Journal of Preventive Cardiology* (December 2014).

34. Vizcaino, M. "Hatha yoga practice for type 2 diabetes mellitus patients: a pilot study." *International Journal of Yoga Therapy* 23 (2013): 59-65.

35. Chimkode, S. M., S. D. Kumaran, V. V. Kanhere, and R. Shivanna. "Effect of yoga on blood glucose levels in patients with type 2 diabetes." *Journal of Clinical and Diagnostic Research* 9 (April 2015): CC01-3.

36. Davis, K., S. H. Goodman, J. Leiferman, M. Taylor, and S. Dimidjian. "A randomized controlled trial of yoga for pregnant women with symptoms of depression and anxiety." *Complementary Therapies in Clinical Practice* 21 (August 2015): 166-172.

37. Curtis, K., A. Weinrib, and J. Katz. "Systematic review of yoga for pregnant women: current status and future directions." *Evidence-Based Complementary and Alternative Medicine* (2012).

38. Chuntharapat, S., W. Petpichetchian, and U. Hatthakit. "Yoga during pregnancy: effect on maternal comfort, labor pain and birth outcome." *Complementary Therapies in Clinical Practice* 14 (May 2008): 105-115.

39. Rakhshani, Abbas, Raghuram Nagarathna, Rita Mhaskar, Arun Mhaskar, Annamma Thomas, and Sulochana Gunasheela. "Effect of Yoga on Utero-Fetal-Placental Circulation in High-Risk Pregnancy: a

Randomized Controlled Trial." *Advances in Preventive Medicine* (January 2015): 373041.

40. Sudarshan, M., A. Petrucci, S. Dumitra, J. Duplisea, S. Wexler, and S. Meterissian. "Yoga therapy for breast cancer patients: a prospective cohort study." *Complementary Therapies in Clinical Practice* 19 (November 2013): 227-229.

41. Peppone, L. J., M. C. Janelsins, C. Kamen, S. G. Mohile, et al. "The effect of YOCAS yoga for musculoskeletal symptoms among breast cancer survivors on hormonal therapy." *Breast Cancer Research and Treatment* 150 (April 2015): 597-604.

42. Mustian, K. M. "Yoga as treatment for insomnia among cancer patients and survivors: a systematic review." *European Medical Journal: Oncology* 1 (November 2013): 106-115.

43. Sodhi, C., S. Singh, and A. Bery. "Assessment of the quality of life in patients with bronchial asthma before and after yoga: a randomized trial." *Iranian Journal of Allergy, Asthma, and Immunology* 13 (February 2014): 55-60.

44. Agnihotri, S., S. Kant, S. Kumar, R. K. Mishra, and S. K. Mishra. "Impact of yoga on biochemical profile of asthmatics: a randomized controlled study." *International Journal of Yoga* 7 (January 2014): 17-21.

45. Fulambarker, A., B. Farooki, F. Kheir, A. S. Copur, L. Srinivason, and S. Schultz. "Effect of yoga in chronic obstructive pulmonary disease." *American Journal of Therapeutics* 19 (March 2012): 96-100.

46. Liu, X. C., L. Pan, Q. Hu, W. P. Dong, J. H. Yan, and L. Dong. "Effects of yoga training in patients with chronic obstructive pulmonary disease: a systematic review and meta-analysis." *Journal of Thoracic Disease* 6 (June 2014): 795-802.

47. Frank, R., and J. Larimore. "Yoga as a method of symptom management in multiple sclerosis." *Frontiers in Neuroscience* 9 (April 2015): 133.

48. Guner, S., and F. Inanici. "Yoga therapy and ambulatory multiple sclerosis assessment of gait analysis parameters, fatigue and balance." *Journal of Bodywork and Movement Therapies* 19 (January 2015): 72-81.
49. Dehkordi, A. Hassanpour. "Influence of yoga and aerobic exercise on fatigue, pain and psychosocial status in patients with multiple sclerosis: a randomized trial." *The Journal of Sports Medicine and Physical Fitness* (July 2015).
50. Khalsa, S. B. "Treatment of chronic insomnia with yoga: a preliminary study with sleep wake diaries." *Applied Psychophysiology and Biofeedback* 29 (December 2004): 269-278.
51. Halpern, J., M. Cohen, G. Kennedy, J. Reece, C. Cahan, and A. Baharav. "Yoga for improving sleep quality and quality of life for older adults." *Alternative Therapies in Health and Medicine* 20 (May-June 2014): 37-46.
52. Chen, K. M., M. H. Chen, M. H. Lin, J. T. Fan, H. S. Lin, and C. H. Li. "Effects of yoga on sleep quality and depression in elderly in assisted living facilities." *The Journal of Nursing Research* 18 (March 2010): 53-61.
53. Afonso, R. F., H. Hachul, E. H. Kozasa, Dde S. Oliveira, V. Goto, D. Rodrigues, S. Tufik, and J. R. Leite. "Yoga decreases insomnia in postmenopausal women: a randomized clinical trial." *Menopause* 19 (February 2012): 186-193.
54. Avis, N. E., C. Legault, G. Russell, K. Weaver, and S. C. Danhauer. "Pilot study of integral yoga for menopausal hot flashes." *Menopause* 21 (August 2014): 846-854.
55. Cohen, B. E. "Yoga: an evidence based prescription for menopausal symptoms?" *Menopause* 15 (Sep-Oct 2008): 827-829.
56. Elibero, A., K. Janse Van Rensburg, and D. J. Drobes. "Acute effects of aerobic exercise and hatha yoga on craving to smoke." *Nicotine & Tobacco Research* 13 (November 2011): 1140-1148.

57. Hallgren, M., K. Romberg, A. S. Bakshi, and S. Andreasson. "Yoga as an adjunct treatment for alcohol dependance: a pilot study." *Complementary Therapies in Medicine* 22 (June 2014): 441-445.

58. Holton, M. K., and A. E. Barry. "Do side effects/ injuries from yoga practice result in discontinued use?" *International Journal of Yoga* 7 (July 2014): 152-154.

59. Russell, K., S. Gushue, S. Richmond, and S. McFaull. "Epidemiology of yoga related injuries in Canada from 1991 to 2010: a case series study." *International Journal of Injury Control and Safety Promotion* 23 (September 2016).

60. Ferrera, C., M. Echavarria-Pinto, I. Nunez-Gil, and F. Alfonso. "Bikram yoga and acute myocardial infarction" *Journal of the American College of Cardiology* 63 (April 2014): 1223.

61. Woodyard, C. "Exploring the therapeutic effects of yoga and its ability to increase quality of life." *International Journal of Yoga* 4 (July-Dec 2011): 49-54.

62. Verrastro, G. "Yoga as therapy: when it is helpful?" *The Journal of Family Practice* 63 (September 2014): E1-6.

Chapter 5

1. Pitocco, D, F. Zaccardi, E. Di Stasio, F. Romitelli, S. A. Santini, C. Zuppi, and G. Ghirlanda. "Oxidative stress, nitric oxide and diabetes." *The Review of Diabetic Studies* 7 (Spring 2010): 15-25.

2. Cohen, S., D. Janicki-Deverts, and G. Miller. "Psychological stress and disease." *Journal of American Medical Association* 298 (October 2007): 1685-1687.

3. McIntosh, L. J. and R. M. Sapolsky. "Glucocorticoids may enhance oxygen radical mediated neurotoxicity." *Neurotoxicology* 17 (Fall-Winter 1996): 873-882.

4. Sharma, M. and S. E. Rush. "Mindfulness-based reduction as a stress management intervention for health

individuals." *Journal of Evidence-Based Complementary and Alternative Medicine* 19 (October 2014) 271-286.

5. Goyal, M., S. Singh, E. M. Sibinga, N. F. Gould, et al. "Meditation programs for psychological stress and well-being: a systematic review and meta-analysis." *Journal of American Medical Association: Internal Medicine* 174 (March 2014): 357-368.
6. Elder, C., S. Nidich, F. Moriarty, and R. Nidich. "Effect of transcendental meditation on employee stress, depression and burnout: a randomized controlled study." *The Permanente Journal* 18 (Winter 2014): 19-23.
7. Kemper, K. J., D. Powell, C. C. Helms, and D. B. Kim-Shapiro. "Loving-kindness meditation's effect on nitric oxide and perceived well-being: a pilot study in experienced and inexperienced meditators." *Explore* 11 (Jan-Feb 2015): 32-39.
8. Hoffman, S. G., P. Grossman, and D. E. Hinton. "Loving-kindness and compassion meditation: potential for psychological interventions." *Clinical Psychology Review* 31 (November 2011): 1126-1132.
9. Bormann, J. E., T. L. Smith, S. Becker, M. Gershwin, L. Pada, A. H. Grudzinski, and E. A. Nurmi. "Efficacy of frequent mantra repetition on stress, quality of life and spiritual well-being in veterans: a pilot study." *Journal of Holistic Nursing* 23 (December 2005): 395-314.
10. Borman, J. E., D. Oman, J. K. Kemppainen, S. Becker, M. Gershwin, and A. Kelly. "Mantram repetition for stress management in veterans and employees: a critical incident study." *Journal of Advanced Nursing* 53 (March 2006): 502-512.
11. Turakitwanakan, W., C. Mekseepralard, and P. Busarakumtragul. "Effects of mindfulness meditation on serum cortisol of medical students." *Journal of the Medical Association of Thailand* 96 Supply 1 (January 2013): S90-95.
12. Brand, S., E. Holsboer-Trachsler, R. Naranjo, S. Schmidt. "Influence of mindfulness practice on cortisol and sleep in

long term and short term meditators." *Neuropsychobiology* 65 (2012): 109-118.

13. Walton, K. G., J. Z. Fields, D. K. Levitsky, D. A. Harris, N. D. Pugh, and R. H. Schneider. "Lowering cortisol and CVD risk in postmenopausal women: a pilot study using transcendental meditation program." *Annals of the New York Academy of Sciences* 1032 (December 2004): 211-215.
14. Mahagita, C. "Roles of meditation on alleviation of oxidative stress and improvement of antioxidant system." *Journal of the Medical Association of Thailand* 93 Supply 6 (November 2010): S242-254.
15. Kim, D. H., Y. S. Moon, H. S. Kim, J. S. Jung, H. M. Suh, Y. H. Kim, and D. K. Song. "Effect of Zen meditation on serum nitric oxide activity and lipid peroxidation." *Progress in Neuro-Psychopharmacology & Biological Psychiatry* 29 (February 2005): 327-331.
16. Orme-Johnson, D. "Medical care utilization and the transcendental meditation program." *Psychosomatic Medicine* 49 (Sep-Oct, 1987): 493-507.
17. Herron, R. E. "Changes in physician costs among high-cost transcendental meditation practitioners compared with high cost non practitioners over 5 years." *American Journal of Health Promotion* 26 (Sept-Oct 2011): 56-60.
18. Walton, K., R. H. Schneider, and S. Nidich. "Review of controlled research on the transcendental meditation program and cardiovascular disease: risk factors, morbidity and mortality." *Cardiology in Review* 12 (Sep-Oct 2004): 262-266.
19. Koika, M. K. and R. Cardoso. "Meditation can produce beneficial effects to prevent cardiovascular disease." *Hormone Molecular Biology and Clinical Investigation* 18 (June 2014): 137-143.
20. Dobos, G., T. Overhamm, A. Bussing, T. Ostermann, J. Langhorst, S. Kummel, A. Paul, and H. Cramer. "Integrating mindfulness in supportive cancer care: a cohort study on a mindfulness-based day care clinic

for cancer survivors." *Supportive Care in Cancer* 23 (October 2015).

21. Robb, Sara Wagner, Kelsey Benson, Lauren Middleton, Christine Meyers, and James R. Hebert. "Mindfulness based stress reduction teachers, practice characteristics, cancer incidence and health: a nationwide ecological description." *BioMed Central Complementary and Alternative Medicine* 15 (February 2015): 24

22. Anderson, J. W., C. Liu, R. J. Kryscio. "Blood pressure response to transcendental meditation: a meta-analysis." *American Journal of Hypertension* 21 (March 2008): 310-316.

23. Rosenzweig, S., D. K. Reibel, J. M. Greeson, J. S. Edman, S. A. Jasser, K. D. McMEarty, and B. J. Goldstein. "Mindfulness-based stress reduction is associated with improved glycemic control in typer-2 diabetes mellitus: a pilot study." *Alternative Therapies in Health and Medicine* 13 (Sep-Oct 2007): 36-38.

24. Chaiopanont, S. "Hypoglycemic effect of sitting breathing meditation exercise on type 2 diabetes in Wat Khae Nok primary health care center in Nonthaburi province." *Journal of the Medical Association of Thailand* 91 (January 2008): 93-98.

25. Solberg, E. E., R. Halvorsen, J. Sundgot-Borgen, F. Ingier, and A. Holen. "Meditation: a modulator of the immune response to physical exercise? A brief report." *British Journal of Sports Medicine* 29 (December 1995): 255-257.

26. Morgan, N., M. R. Irwain, M. Chung, and C. Wang. "The effect of mind-body therapies on the immune system: metaanalysis." *PLoS One* 9 (July 2014): e100903.

27. Kiran, K. K Girgla, H. Chalana, and H. Singh. "Effect of raja-yoga meditation on chronic tension headache." *Indian Journal of Physiology and Pharmacology* 58 (April-June 2014): 157-161.

28. Wells, R. E., R. Burch, R. H. Paulsen, P. M. Wayne, T. T. Houle, and E. Loder. "Meditation for migraines: a pilot

randomized controlled trial." *Headache* 54 (October 2014): 1484-1495.

29. Reiner, K., L. Tibi, and J. D. Lipsitz. "Do mindfulness-based interventions reduce pain intensity? A critical review of literature." *Pain Medicine* 14 (February 2013): 230-242.
30. Ia Cour, P., M. Petersen. "Effects of mindfulness meditation on chronic pain: a randomized clinical trial." *Pain Medicine* 16 (April 2015): 641-652.
31. Morone, N. E., C. S. Lynch, C. M. Greco, H. A. Tindle, and D. K. Weiner. "'I felt like a new person' the effects of mindfulness meditation on older adults with chronic pain: qualitative narrative analysis of diary entries." *The Journal of Pain* 9 (September 2008): 841-848.
32. Black, D. S., G. A. O'Reilly, R. Olmstead, E. C. Breen, and M. R. Irwin. "Mindfulness meditation and improvement in sleep quality and daytime impairment among older adults with sleep disturbances: a randomized clinical trial." *Journal of American Medical Association: Internal Medicine* 175 (April 2015): 494-501.
33. Ong, J. C., R. Manber, Z. Segal, Y. Xia, S. Shapiro, and J. K. Wyatt. "A randomized controlled trial of mindfulness meditation for chronic insomnia." *Sleep* 37 (September 2014): 1553-1563.
34. Sun, J., J. Kang, P. Wang, and H. Zeng. "Self-relaxation training can improve sleep quality and cognitive functions in the older adults: a one year randomized controlled trial." *Journal of Clinical Nursing* 22 (May 2013): 1270-1280.
35. Kurth, F., N. Cherbuin, and E. Luders. "Reduced age-related degeneration in the hippocampal subiculum in long term meditators." *Psychiatry Research* 232 (June 2015): 214-218.
36. Hoge, Elizabeth A., Maxin M. Chen, Ester Orr, Christina A. Metcalf, Laura E. Fischer, Mark Pollack, Immaculata, Devivo, and Miklos Dezxo Simon. "Loving kindness meditation practice associated with longer telomeres

in women." *Brain Behavior and Immunity* 32 (April 2013): 159-163.

37. Alexander, C. N., E. J. Langer, R. I. Newman, H. M. Chandler, and J. L. Davies. "Transcendental meditation, mindfulness and longevity: an experimental study with elderly." *Journal of Personality and Social Psychology* 57 (December 1989): 950-964.
38. Xiong, G. L. and P. M. Doraiswamy. "Does meditation enhance cognition and brain plasticity." *Annals of the New York Academy of Sciences* 1172 (August 2009): 63-69.
39. Luders, E., F. Kurth, E. A. Mayer, A. W. Toga, K. L. Narr, and C. Gaser. "The unique brain anatomy of meditation practitioners: alteration in cortical gyrification." *Frontiers in Human Neuroscience* 6 (February 2012): 34.
40. Holzel, Britta K., James Carmody, Mark Vanger, Christina Congleton, Sita M. Yerramsetti, Tim Gard, and Sara W. Lazar. "Mindfulness practice leads to increases in regional brain gray matter." *Psychiatry Research* 191 (January 2011): 36-43.
41. Posner, Michael I., Yi-Yuan Tang, and Gary Lynch. "Mechanism of white matter change induced by meditation training." *Frontiers in Psychology* 5 (October 2014): 1220.
42. Jindal, V., S. Gupta, and R. Das. "Molecular mechanism of meditation." *Molecular Neurobiology* 48 (December 2013): 808-811.
43. Miller, K. M., E. Chad-Friedman, V. Haime, D. H. Mehta, et al. "The effectiveness of a brief mind-body intervention for treating depression in community health center patients." *Clobal Advances in Health and Medicine* 4 (March 2015): 30-35.
44. Greeson, J. M., M. J. Smoski, E. C. Suarez, J. G. Brantley, A. G. Ekblad, T. R. Lynch, and R. Q. Wolever. "Decreased symptoms of depression after mindfulnessbased stress reduction: potential moderating effects of religiosity, spirituality, trait mindfulness, sex and age." *Journal of*

Alternative and Complementary Medicine 21 (March 2015): 1660174.

45. Kearney, D. J., C. A. Malte, C. McManus, M. E. Martinez, B. Felleman, and T. L. Simpson. "Loving-kindness meditation for posttraumatic stress disorder: a pilot study." *Journal of Traumatic Stress* 26 (August 2013): 426-434.
46. Himelstein, Samuel. "Meditation research: the state of the art in correctional settings." *International Journal of Offender Therapy and Comparative Criminology* 60 (September 2016): 646-661.
47. Luders, E. "Exploring age-related brain degeneration in meditation practitioners." *Annals of the New York Academy of Sciences* 1307 (January 2014): 82-88.
48. Tang, Y. Y., R. Tang, M. I. Posner. "Brief meditation training induces smoking reduction." *Proceedings of the National Academy of Sciences in the United States of America* 110 (August 2013): 13971-13975.
49. Shafil, M., R. Lavely, and R. Jaffe. "Meditation and prevention of alcohol use." *American Journal of Psychiatry* 132 (October 1975): 942-945.
50. Black, David S. "Mindfulness and substance use intervention." *Substance Use & Misuse* (January 2012): 199-201.
51. Aron, A. and E. N. Aron. "The transcendental meditation program's effect on addictive behavior." *Addictive Behaviors* 5 (1980): 3-12.
52. Chen, K. W., A. Comerford, P. Shinnick, and D. M. Ziedonis. "Introducing qigong meditation into residential addiction treatment: a pilot study where gender makes a difference." *Journal of Alternative and Complementary Medicine* 16 (August 2010): 875-882.
53. Kristeller, Jean L. and C. Brendan Hallet. "An exploratory study of a meditation based intervention for binge eating disorder." *Journal of Health Psychology* 4 (May 1999): 357-363.

54. Katterman, S. N., B. M. Kleinman, M. M. Hood, L. M. Nackers, and J. A. Corsica. "Mindfulness meditation as an intervention for binge eating, emotional eating and weight loss." *Eating Behaviors* 15 (April 2014): 197-204.

55. Lagopoulos, J., J. Xu, I. Rasmussen, A. Vik, et al. "Increased theta and alpha EEG activity during nondirective meditation." *Journal of Alternative and Complementary Medicine* 15 (November 2009): 1187-1192.

56. Pasquini, Henrique Adam, Ken Tanaka, Luis Fernando Hindi Basile, Bruna Velasques, Mirna Delposo Lozano, and Pedro Ribeiro. "Electrophysiological correlates of long term Soto-Zen meditation." *BioMed Research International* (January 2015): 598496.

57. Tsai, J. F., S. H. Jou, W. Cho, and C. M. Li. "Electroencephalography when meditation advances: a case based time series analysis." *Cognitive Processing* 14 (November 2013): 371-376.

58. Travis, Frederick. "Transcendental experiences during meditation practice." *Annals of the New York Academy of Sciences* 1307 (March 2014): 1-8.

59. Mason, L. I., C. N. Alexander, F. T. Travis, G. Marsh, D. W. Orme-Johnson, J. Gackenbach, D. C. Mason, M. Rainforth, and K. G. Walton. "Electrophysiological correlates of higher state of consciousness during sleep in long term practitioners of transcendental meditation." *Sleep* 20 (February 1997): 102-110.

60. Lutz, A., L. L. Greischar, N. B. Rawlings, M. Ricard, and R. J. Davidson. "Long term meditators self-induced high amplitude synchrony during mental practice." *Proceedings of the National Academy of Sciences of the United States of America* 101 (November 2004): 16369-16373.

61. Kjaer, T. W., C. Bertelsen, P. Piccini, D. Brooks, J. Alving, and H. C. Lou. "Increased dopamine tone during meditation-induced change in consciousness." *Brain Research: Cognitive Brain Research* 13 (April 2002): 255-259.

Chapter 6

1. Ikedo, F., D. M. Gangahar, M. A. Quader, and L. M. Smith. "The effects of prayer, relaxation technique during general anesthesia on recovery outcomes following cardiac surgery." *Complementary Therapies in Clinical Practice* 13 (May 2007): 85-94.
2. Saudia, T. L., M. R. Kinney, K. C. Brown, and L. Young-Ward. "Health locus of control and helpfulness of prayer." *Heart & Lung, the Journal of Critical Care* 20 (January 1991): 60-65.
3. Richardson, M. A., T. Sanders, J. L. Plamer, A. Greisinger A, and S. E. Singletary. "Complementary/alternative medicine use in a comprehensive cancer center and implications for oncology." *Journal of Clinical Oncology* 18 (July 2000): 2505-2514.
4. Jors, K., A. Bussing, N. C. Hvidt, and K. Baumann. "Personal prayer in patients dealing with chronic illness: a review of the research literature." *Evidence-Base Complementary and Alternative Medicine* (2015): 927973.
5. Byrd, R. C. "Positive therapeutic effects of intercessory prayer in a coronary care unit population." *Southern Medical Journal* 81 (July 1988): 826-829.
6. Harris, W. S., M. Gowda, J. W. Kolb, C. P. Strychacz, J. L. Vacek, P. G. Jones, A. Forker, J. H. O-Keefe, and B. D. McCallister. "A randomized controlled trial of the effects of remote intercessory prayer on outcomes in patients admitted to the coronary care unit." *Archives of Internal Medicine* 159 (October 1999): 2273-2278.
7. Leibovici, L. "Effects of remote retroactive intercessory prayer on outcomes in patients with blood stream infection: randomized controlled trial." *British Medical Journal* 323 (December 2001): 1450-1451.
8. Metthews, D. A., S. M. Marlowe, and F. S. MacNutts. "Effects of intercessory prayer on patients with rheumatoid arthritis."

9. *Southern Medical Journal* 93 (December 2000): 1177-1186.
10. Vannemreddy, P., K. Bryan, and A. Nanda. "Influence of prayer and prayer habits on outcome in patients with severe head injury." *The American Journal of Hospice and Palliative Care* 26 (Aug-Sep 2009): 264-269.
11. Ratnasingam, D., D. S. Lovick, D. M. Weber, R. V. Buonocore, and W. V. Williams. "An usual recovery from traumatic brain injury in a young man." *The Linacre Quarterly* 82 (February 2015): 55-66.
12. Hughes, Christina E. "Prayer and healing: a case study." *Journal of Holistic Nursing* 15 (October 1997): 318-324.
13. Olver, I. N., and A. Dutney. "A randomized blinded study of the impact of intercessory prayer on spiritual well-being in patients with cancer." *Alternative Therapies in Health and Medicine* 18 (Sep-Oct 2012): 18-27.
14. Coruh, B., H. Ayele, M. Pugh, and T. Mulligan. "Does religious activity improve health outcome? A critical review of the recent literature." *Explore* 1 (May 2005): 186-191.
15. Robets, L., I. Ahmed, S. Hall, C. Sargent, and C. Adams. "Intercessory prayer for ill health: a systematic review." *Forschende Komplementarmedizin* 5 Supply 1 (1998): 82-86.
16. Benson, H., J. A. Dusek, B. Sherwood, P. Lam, et al. "Study of the therapeutic effect of intercessory prayer (STEP) in cardiac bypass patients: a multicenter randomized trial of uncertainty or receiving intercessory prayer." *American Heart Journal* 151 (April 2006): 934-942.
17. Roberts, L., I. Ahmed, S. Hall, and A. Davison. "Intercessory prayer for the alleviation of ill health." *The Cochrane Database of Systematic Reviews* (April 2009): CD000368.
18. Walker, S. R., J. S. Tonigan, W. R. Miller, S. Corner, and L. Kahlich. "Intercessory prayer in the treatment of alcohol abuse and dependence: a pilot investigation." *Alternative Therapies in Health and Medicine* 3 (November 1997): 79-86.

19. Mathai, J. and A. Bourne. "Pilot study investigating the effect of intercessory prayer in the treatment of child psychiatric disorders." *Australiasian Psychiatry* 12 (December 2004): 386-389.

20. Nosky, B., J. Min, V. D. Lima, B. Yip, R. S. Hoggs, and J. S. Montaner. "HIV-1 disease progression during highly active antiretroviral therapy: an application using population-level data in British Columbia: 1996-2011." *Journal of Acquired Immune Deficiency Syndromes* 63 (August 2013):653-659.

21. Astin, J. A., J. Stone, D. I. Abrams, D. H. Moore, P. Couey, R. Buscemi, and E. Targ. "The efficacy of distant healing for human immunodeficiency virus—results of a randomized trial." *Alternative Therapies in Health and Medicine* 12 (Nov-Dec 2006): 36-41.

22. Ironson, G. and H. Kremer. "Spiritual transformation, psychological well-being, health and survival in people with HIV." *International Journal of Psychiatry and Medicine* 39 (2009): 263-281.

23. Kremer, H., G. Ironson, L. Kaplan, R. Stuetzele, N. Baker, and M. A. Fletcher. "Spritual coping predicts CD4 cell preservation and undetectable viral load over four years." *AIDS Care* 27 (2015): 71-79.

24. Ironson, G., R. Stuetzle, D. Ironson, E. Balbin, H. Kremer, A. George, N. Schneiderman, and M. A. Fletcher. "View of God as benevolent and forgiving or punishing and judgemental predicts HIV disease progression." *Journal of Behavioral Medicine* 34 (December 2011): 414-425.

25. Cha, K. Y. and D. P. Writh. "Does prayer influence the success of in vitro fertilization-embryo transfer? Report of a masked, randomized trial." *The Journal of Reproductive Medicine* 46 (September 2001): 781-787.

26. Bhasin, M. K., J. A. Dusel, B. H. Chang, M. G. Joseph, J. W. Denninger, G. L. Fricchione, H. Benson, and T. A. Libermann. "Relaxation responses induce temporal transcriptome changes in energy metabolism, insulin

secretion and inflammatory pathways." *PLoS One* 8 (May 2013): e62817.

27. Lutgendrof, S. K., D. Russel, P. Ullrich, T. B. Harris, and R. Wallace. "Religious participation, interleukin-6 and mortality in older adults." *Health Psychology* 23 (September 2004): 465-475.
28. Mody, B. S. "Acute effects of Surya Namaskar on the cardiovascular and metabolic system." *Journal of Bodywork and Movement Therapies* 15 (July 2011): 343-347.
29. Koeing, H. G. "An 83 year old woman with chronic illness and strong religious beliefs." *Journal of American Medical Association* 288 (July 2002): 487-493.
30. Leder, D. "Spooky action at distance" physics, psi, and distant healing." *Journal of Alternative and Complementary Medicine* 11 (October 2005): 923-930.
31. Rading, D. I. "Event related electroencephalographic correlations between isolated human subjects." *Journal of Alternative and Complementary Medicine* 10 (April 2004): 315-323.
32. Toms, R. "Reiki therapy: a nursing intervention for critical care." *Critical Care Nursing Quarterly* 34 (July-Sep 2011): 213-217.
33. Rosade, R. M., B. Rubik, B. Mainguy, J. Plummer, L. Mehl-Madrona. "Reiki reduces burnout among community mental health clinicians." *Journal of Alternative and Complementary Medicine* 21 (August 2015): 489-495.
34. Bukowski, E. L. and D. Berardi. "Reiki brief report: using Reiki to reduce stress levels in a nine year old child." *Explore* 10 (July-Aug 2014): 253-255.
35. Olson, K., J. Hanson, and A. Michaud. "A phase II trial of Reiki for the management of pain in advanced cancer patients." *Journal of Pain and Symptom Management* 26 (November 2006): 990-97.

36. Bullock, M. "Reiki: a complementary therapy for life." *The American Journal of Hospice & Palliative Care* 14 (Jan-Feb 1997): 31-33.

37. Gillespie, E. A., B. W. Gillespie, and M. J. Stevens. "Painful diabetic neuropathy: impact on an alternative approach." *Diabetes Care* 30 (April 2007): 999-1001.

38. Vitale, A., and P. O'Conner. "The effect of Reiki on pain and anxiety in women with abdominal hysterectomies: a quasi-experimental pilot study." *Holistic Nursing Practice* 20 (Nov-Dec 2006): 263-274.

39. Demir, M., G. Can, A. Kelam, and A. Aydiner. "Effects of distant Reiki on pain, anxiety and fatigue in oncology patients in Turkey: a pilot study." *Asian Pacific Journal of Cancer Prevention* 16 (2015): 4849-1862.

40. Joyce, J., and G. P. Herbison. "Reiki for depression and anxiety." *The Cochrane Database of Systematic Reviews* (April 2015): CD006833.

41. Wong, J., A. Ghiasuddin, C. Kimata, B. Patelesio, and A. Siu. "The impact of healing touch on pediatric oncology patients." *Integrative Cancer Therapies* 12 (January 2013): 25-30.

42. Decker, S., D. W. Wardell, and S. G. Cron. "Using a healing touch intervention in older adults with persistent pain: a feasibility study." *Journal of Holistic Nursing* 30 (September 2012): 205-213.

43. Lincoln, V., E. W. Nowak, B. Schommer, T. Briggs, A Fehrer, and G. Wax. "Impact of healing touch with healing harp on inpatient acute pain: a retrospective analysis." *Holistic Nursing Practice* 28 (May-June 2014): 164-170.

44. Lu, D. F., L. K. Hart, S. K. Lutgendorf, and Y. Perkhounkova. "The effect of healing touch on the pain and mobility of persons with osteoarthritis: a feasibility study." *Geriatric Nursing* 34 (July-Aug 2013): 314-322.

45. Wetzel, W. S. "Healing touch as a nursing intervention: wound infection following cesarean birth-an anecdotal

study." *Journal of Holistic Nursing* 11 (September 1993): 277-285.

46. Goldberger, D. R., D. W. Wardell, N. Kilgarriff, B. Williams, D. Eichler, and P. Thomlinson. "An initial study using healing touch for women undergoing a breast biopsy." *Journal of Holistic Nursing* 34 (June 2016).
47. Anderson, J. G., L. Suchicital, M. Lang, A. Kukic, L. Mangione, D. Swengros, J. Fabian, and M. A. Friesen. "The effects of healing touch on pain, nausea, and anxiety following bariatric surgery: a pilot study." *Explore* 11 (May-June 2015): 208-216.
48. Umbreit, A. W. "Healing touch: applications in the acute care setting." *AACN Clinical Issues* 11 (February 2000): 105-119.
49. Schlitz, M., H. W. Hopf, L. Eskenazi, C. Vieten, and D. Radin. "Distant healing of surgical wounds: an exploratory study." *Explore* 8 (July-Aug 2012): 223-230.
50. Sicher, F., E. Targ, D. Moore 2nd, H. S. Smith. "A randomized double blind study of the effect of distant healing in population with advanced AIDS. Report of a small scale study." *The Western Journal of Medicine* 169 (December 1998): 356-363.
51. Astin, J. A., E. Harkness, and E. Ernst. "The efficacy of distant healing: a systematic review of randomized trials." *Annals of Internal Medicine* 132 (June 2000): 903-910.
52. Walach, H., H. Bosch, G. Lewith, J. Naumann, et al. "Effectiveness of distant healing for patients with chronic fatigue syndrome: a randomized controlled partially blinded trial (EUHEALS)." *Psychotherapy and Psychosomatics* 77 (2008): 158-166.
53. Meissner, K. and A. Koch. "Sympathetic arousal during a touch based healing ritual predicts increased well-being." *Evidence-Based complementary and Alternative Medicine* (July 2015).

Chapter 7

1. Diener, E., S. Oishi, and R. E. Lucas. "Personality, culture and subjective well-being: emotional and cognitive evaluations of life." *Annual Review of Psychology* 54 (2003): 403-425.
2. Layard, R. "Measuring subjective well-being." *Science Magazine* 327 (January 2010): 534-535.
3. Oishi, Shigehiro and Selin Kesebir. "Income inequality explains why economic growth does not always translates to an increase in happiness." *Psychological Science* (October 2015).
4. Mogilner, C. "The pursuit of happiness: time, money and social connection." *Psychological Science* 21 (September 2010): 1348-1354.
5. Quoidbach, J., E. W. Dunn, K. V. Petrides, and M. Mikolajczak. "Money giveth, money taketh away: the dual effect of wealth on happiness." *Psychological Science* 21 (June 2010): 759-763.
6. Dunn, E. W., L. B. Aknin, and M. I. Norton. "Spending money on others promotes happiness." *Science* 319 (March 2008): 1687-1688.
7. Kehneman, D. and A. Deaton. "High income improves evaluation of life but not emotional well-being." *Proceedings of the National Academy of Sciences of the United States of America* 107 (September 2010): 16489-16493.
8. Taylor, S. E., L. C. Klein, B. P. Lewis, T. L. Gruenewald, R. A. Gurung, and J. A. Updegraff. "Biobehavioral response to stress in females: tend and befriend, not fight or flight." *Psychological Review* 107 (2000): 411-429.
9. McDaniel, B. T., S. M. Coyne, and E. K. Holmes. "New mothers and media use: associations between blogging, social networking and maternal wellbeing." *Maternal and Child Health Journal* 16 (October 2012): 1509-1517.
10. Olstad, R., H. Sexton, and A. J. Sogaard. "The Finnmark study: a prospective population study of the social support

buffer hypothesis, specific stressors and mental distress." *Social Psychiatry and Psychiatric Epidemiology* 36 (December 2001): 582-589.

11. Wooten, P. "Humor: an antidote for stress." *Holistic Nursing Practice* 10 (January 1996): 49-56.
12. Wells, Deborah L. "The facilitation of social interactions by domestic dogs." *Anthrozoos* 17 (January 2004): 340-352.
13. Odendaal, J. S. and R. A. Meintjes. "Neurophysiological correlation of affiliative behavior between humans and dogs." *Veterinary Journal* 165 (May 2003): 296-301.
14. Woodcock, J., O. H. Franco, N. Orsini, and I. Roberts. "Non-vigorous physical activity and all-cause mortality: systematic review and meta-analysis of cohort studies." *International Journal of Epidemiology* 40 (February 2011): 121-138.
15. Haskell, W. L., I. M. Lee, R. R. Pate, K. E. Powell, et al. "Physical activity and public health: updated recommendation for adults from the American College of Sports Medicine and the American Heart Association." *Medicine and Science in Sports and Exercise* 39 (August 2007): 1423-1434.
16. Atsumi, T, and K. Tonosaki. "Smelling lavender and rosemary increases free radical scavenging activity and decreases cortisol level in saliva." *Psychiatry Research* 150 (February 2007): 89-96.
17. Labrique-Walusis, F., K. J. Keister, and A. C. Russell. "Massage therapy for stress management: implications for nursing practice." *Orthopedic Nursing* 29 (July-Aug 2010): 254-257.
18. Cervellin, G. and G. Lippi. "From music beat to heart beat: a journey in the complex interactions between music, brain and heart." *European Journal of Internal Medicine* 22 (August 2011): 371-374.
19. Burleson, M. H., W. R. Trevathan, and M. Todd. "In the mood for love or vice versa? Exploring the relations among sexual activity, physical affection, affect and stress in the

daily lives of mid-aged women." *Archives of Sexual Behavior* 36 (June 2007): 357-368.

20. Gump, B. B. and K. A. Matthews. "Are vacations good for your health? The 9-year mortality experience after the multiple risk factors intervention trail." *Psychosomatic Medicine* 62 (Sep-Oct 2000): 608-612.
21. Woodyard, C. "Exploring the therapeutic effects of yoga and its ability to increase quality of life." *International Journal of Yoga* 4 (July-Dec 2011): 49-54.
22. Hartfiel, N., J. Havenhand, S. B. Khalsa, G. Clarke, and A. Krayer. "The effectiveness of yoga for the improvement of well-being and resilience to stress in the workplace." *Scandinavian Journal of Work, Environment and Health* 37 (January 2011): 70-76.
23. Sharma, R., N. Gupta, and R. Bijlani. "Effect of yoga based lifestyle intervention on subjective well-being." *Indian Journal of Physiology and Pharmacology* 52 (April-June 2008): 123-131.
24. Malathi, A., A. Damodaran, N. Shah, N. Patil, and S. Maratha. "Effect of yoga practices on subjective well-being." *Indian Journal of Physiology and Pharmacology* 44 (April 2000): 202-206.
25. Ivtzan, I., and A. Papantonious. "Yoga meets positive psychology: examining the integration of hedonic (gratitude) and eudaemonic (meaning) wellbeing in relation to the extent of yoga practice." *Journal of Bodywork and Movement Therapies* 18 (April 2014): 183-189.
26. Bussing, Arndt, Anemone Hedstuck, Sat Bir S. Khalsa, Thomas Ostermann, and Peter Heusser. "Development of specific aspects of spirituality during a 6 month intensive yoga practice." *Evidence-Based Complementary and Alternative Medicine* 2012 (2012).
27. Reed, J. "Self-reported morningness-eveningness related to positive affect change associated with a single session of hatha yoga." *International Journal of Yoga Therapy* 24 (2014): 79-85.

28. Streeter, C. C., J. E. Jensen, R. M. Perlmutter, H J. Cabral, H. Tian, D. B. Terhune, D. A. Ciraulo, and P. F. Renshaw. "Yoga asana session increase brain GABA levels: a pilot study." *Journal of Alternative and Complementary Medicine* 13 (May 2007): 419-426.

29. Kamei, T., Y. Toriumi, H. Kimura, S. Ohno, H. Kumano, and K. Kimura. "Decrease in serum cortisol during yoga exercise is correlated with alpha wave activation." *Perceptual and Motor Skills* 90 (June 2000): 1027-1032.

30. Froeliger, Brett E., Eric L. Garland, Leslie A. Modlin, and F. Joseph McClernon. "Neurocognitive correlates of the effects of yoga meditation practice on emotion and cognition: a pilot study." *Frontiers in Integrative Neuroscience* 6 (July 2012): 48.

31. Hills, Peter and Michael Argyle. "The Oxford questionnaire: a compact scale for the measurement of psychological well-being." *Personality Individual Differences* 33 (November 2002): 1073-1082.

32. Ramesh, M. G., B. Sathian, E. Sinu, and K. S. Rai. "Efficacy of rajajoya meditation on positive thinking: an index of selfsatisfaction and happiness in life." *Journal of Clinical and Diagnostic Research* 7 (October 2013): 2265-2267.

33. Brewer, J. A., P. D. Worhunsky, J. R. Gray, Y. Y. Tang, J. Weber, and H. Kober. "Meditation experience is associated with differences in default mode network activity and connectivity." *Proceedings of the National Academy of Sciences of the United States of America* 108 (December 2011): 20254-20259.

34. Tang, Y. Y., Q. Lu, H. Feng, R. Tang, and M. I. Posner. "Short term meditation increases blood flow in the anterior cingulate cortex and insula." *Frontiers in Psychology* 6 (February 2015): 212.

35. Kjaer, T. W., C. Bertselsen, P. Piccini, D. Brooks, J. Alving, and H. C. Lou. "Increased dopamine tone during meditation induced change of consciousness." *Brain Research: Cognitive Brain Research* 13 (April 2002): 255-259.

36. Tkach, Chris and Sonja Lyubomirsky. "How do people pursue happiness? Relating personality, happiness-increasing strategies and well-being." *Journal of Happiness Studies* 7 (February 2006): 183-225.

37. Diener, E., L. Tay, and D. G. Myers. "The religion paradox: if religion makes people happy, why are so many dropping out?" *Journal of Personality and Social Psychology*: 1278-1290.

38. Oishi, Shigehiro, and Ed Diener. "Residents of poor nations have a greater sense of meaning in life than residents of wealthy nations." *Psychological Science* 25 (December 2013): 422-430 and references cited in the paper.

39. Green, M. and M. Elliott. "Religion, health and psychological well-being." *Journal of Religion and Health* 49 (June 2010): 149-163.

40. Berthold, A. and W. Ruch. "Satisfaction with life and character strengths of non-religious and religious people: it's practicing one's religion that makes the difference." *Frontiers in Psychology* 5 (August 2017): 876.

41. Maselko, J. and L. D. Kubzansky. "Gender difference in religious practices, spiritual experiences and health: results from the U.S. general society survey." *Social Science and Medicine* 62 (June 2006): 2848-2860.

42. Vaillant, George E. "Psychiatry, religion, positive emotions and spirituality." *Asian Journal of Psychiatry* 6 (December 2013): 590-594.

43. Barton, Y. A. and L. Liller. "Spirituality and positive psychology go hand in hand: an investigation of multiple empirically derived profiles and related protective benefits." *Journal of Religions and Health* 54 (June 2015): 829-843.

Bonus Section

1. Jones, J. W. and L. B. McCullough. "Medicine versus religion in the surgical intensive care unit: who

is in charge?" *Journal of Vascular Surgery* 57 (April 2013): 1146-1147.

2. Ivy, A. C. "Seven wonders of medical science-modern miracles." *California and Western Medicine* 41 (November 1934): 260-263.
3. Paulson, Steve, Lance Becker, Sam Parnia, and Stephan A. Mayer. "Reversing death: the miracle of modern medicine." *Annals of the New York Academy of Sciences* 1330 (July 2014): 4-18.
4. Sierpina, V. S. "Miracles happen in medicine." *Impact* (December 2013). Accessed February 16, 2015. http://www.utmb.edu/ompact/archive/article. aspx?IAID=1245.
5. Moody, Raymond A. Jr. "Life after Life." Bantam Press, 1975.
6. Moody, Raymond A. Jr. "The Light Beyond." Bantam Press, 1988.
7. Klemenc-Ketis, Z. "Life changes in patients after out-of-hospital cardiac arrest: the effect of near-death experiences." *International Journal of Behavioral Medicine* 20 (March 2013): 7-12.
8. Musella, A., C. Marchetti, L. Salerno, L. Vertechy, R. Iadarola, I. Pecorella, and P. B. Panici. "An unexpected complete remission of advanced intestinal-type vulvar adenocarcinoma after neoadjuvant chemotherapy: a case report and literature review." *Case Reports in Obstetrics and Gynecology* (2013): 427141.
9. Feng, Y. M., C. W. Feng, S. C. Chen, and C. D. Hsu. "Unexpected remission of hepatocellular carcinoma (HCC) with lung metastasis to the combination therapy of thalidomide and cyproheptadine: report of two cases and a preliminary HCC cell line study." *British Medical Journal: Case Reports* (October 2012).
10. Nuzzo, C., M. Zeuli, V. Ferraresi, M. Ciccarese, D. Pelligrini, F. Cognetti. "Unexpected clinical outcome in a patient with liver and brain metastasis from melanoma." *Anticancer Research* 28 (March-April 2008): 1429-1431.

11. Ziegler, J. "Practitioners and saints: medical men in canonization processes in the thirteen to fifteenth centuries." *Social History of Medicine* 12 (August 1999): 191-225.

12. Duffin, J. "The doctor was surprised: or how to diagnose a miracle." *Bulletin of the History of Medicine* 81 (Winter 2007): 699-729.

13. Squires, Nick. "The miracles that earned John Paul II his sainthood," *The Telegraph*, April 23, 2014, http:// www.telegraph.co.uk/news/worldnews/ europe/ vaticancityandholysee/10783125/The-miracle-that-earnedJohn-Paul-II-his-sainthood.html

14. "Reported Miracle Could Make Mother Teresa a Saint." *The Catholic News Agency*, October, 3, 2007. Accessed 2/17/2015, http:www.catholicnewsagency.com/ news/ reported_miracle_could_make_mother_teresa.

15. Francois, Bernard, Esther M. Sternberg, and Elizabeth Fee. "The Lourdes medical cures revisited." *Journal of the History of Medicine and Allied Sciences* 69 (January 2014): 135-162.

16. Martin, J. B. "Miracle on New Year's." *Journal of Christian Nursing* 27 (April-June 2010): 112-113.

17. Nath, Biplab, Pradip Sarkar, and Tapan Das. "Miracle still happens: a rare case of self-inflicted penetrating injury of ear." *Indian Journal of Otolaryngology and Head and Neck Surgery* 66 (January 2014): 107-109.

18. Glod, Susan A. "Miracle". *Journal of American Medical Association: A Piece of My Mind* 311 (April 2014): 1499

19. Broxterman, J. T. "Miracle on 39th street." *Annals of Internal Medicine* 159 (December 2013): 854-855.

20. Kirkpatrick, T. "An old fashioned miracle." *British Medical Journal* 317 (October 1998): 1053C.

21. Morales La Madrid, A. "Waiting for a miracle." *Journal of Clinical Oncology* 30 (July 2012): 2421-2422.

22. Jantos, M. and H. Kiat. "Prayer as medicine: how much have we learned?" *The Medical Journal of Australia* 186 (May 2007): 51-53
23. Ghadirian, A. M. "Is spirituality relevant to the practice of medicine?" *Medicine and Law* 27 (June 2008): 229-233.
24. Slieper, C. F., K. Wasson, and L. M. Ramondetta. "From technician to professional: integrating spirituality into medical practice." *The American Journal of Bioethics* 7 (July 2007): 26-27.
25. Savulescu, J. and S. Clarke. "Waiting for a miracle, miraclism and discrimination." *Southern Medical Journal* 100 (December 2007): 1259-1262.
26. DeLisser, H. "A practical approach to the family that expects a miracle." *Chest* 135 (June 2009): 1643-1647.
27. Cooper, Rhonda S., Anna Ferguson, Joann N. Bodurtha, and Thomas J. Smith. "AMEN in challenging conversations: Bridging the gaps between faith, hope and medicine." *Journal of Oncology Practice* 10 (July 2014): e191-195.
28. Brierley, J., J. Linthicum, and A. Petros. "Should religious beliefs be allowed to stonewall a secular approach to withdrawing and withholding treatment in children?" *Journal of Medical Ethics* 39 (September 2013): 573-577.
29. Pavia, C. E. "When the belief in a miracle is the last thread of hope." *Palliative and Supportive Care* 11 (October 2013): 443-44.